"If it feels like your child's language doesn't follow the usual development pattern, then this is the book for you. Ali provides us with the tools to help our children to develop spontaneous language. My son is one of the children in this book and the joy on his face when he creates new language is something that I treasure. There is so much hope embedded in the GLP approach to speech therapy and it demands that we provide so much more than functional language to our children. Above all though, it allows our children to be children while we are doing it."

Charlotte Beavitt, parent

"Ali's approach is empathic, flexible, sensitive, trusting and fun. With her deep understanding of gestalt processing, she has met our 6-year-old son exactly where he is on his speech development journey. Ali has mindfully equipped us as a family, with the tools and knowledge that benefits us, while not overwhelming us.

"Our son is always so excited to go to 'Ali's house'! for his therapy sessions. There is no doubt, in the words of Barry Prizant, Ali 'gets it'."

Parent

"Ali's book is an absolutely fantastic and accessible resource for parents of Gestalt Language Processors. It's highly informative, clear and detailed and breaks down the complexities of the stages into a comprehensible and practical way. Reading through the chapters resonated with our first-hand experience as parents and was both validating and eye-opening in allowing us to learn and understand more. The use of case studies is especially useful to trace through language samples and understand the different stages of Natural Language Acquisition. Ali is incredibly knowledgeable in this field and her book is a must-have for understanding Gestalt Language Processing and how to provide the right support in a neurodiversity-affirming way."

Michelle, parent

"An essential resource for Speech and Language Therapists, educators and parents, this book on Gestalt Language Processing offers a comprehensive journey through the stages and nuances of how some children acquire language. With its clear explanations, real life case studies, and practical strategies, it empowers readers to feel confident supporting gestalt language development. Ali's depth of knowledge and passion for the subject shines throughout the book. She makes complex theories easy to understand. This book is an invaluable guide for anyone dedicated to supporting Gestalt Language Processors."

Julie Holmes, Speech and Language Therapist

"This book is so positive and detailed. As I read it, I was able to think about and reflect on children I work with. This book encourages our intuition as therapists; to develop a trusting relationship with a child; to allow space, to be in their world and take time to 'get' (understand) them. This has lifted me and made me optimistic for my future support of children who may be GLPs."

Kathryn Seeney, Speech and Language Therapist

"Ali's book has helped me immensely to understand the phenomenon that is Gestalt Language Processing. I knew about GLP previously but was too under-confident to start to really embrace this in my sessions. As a private Speech and Language Therapist, I feel I should 'know it all' to advise my commissioners. Ali's book has made me feel at ease knowing this doesn't have to be the case as I now appreciate, we are ALL still learning about GLP. Ali enables calm reading with her examples and gives excellent practical advice for easy-to-use takeaways."

Becky Sherrington, Speech and Language Therapist

"Such a helpful read! As someone who is new to working with GLP, this book gave me such insight into how everything works and some wonderful ideas on activities to do at each stage. Would highly recommend!"

Maddi English, Speech and Language Therapist

"A comprehensive guide to supporting Gestalt Language Processors, this valuable resource has everything you need to know about working with Gestalt Language Processors and providing support in a neurodiversity affirming way, it explains everything you need to know about GLP in a really accessible way with loads of practical ideas and solutions."

Jess Wates, Speech and Language Therapist

"Ali cuts through a complex set of ideas to make it easily understood by the reader. The easy read format has led me to feel confident in beginning to use the theory with my own clients and keen to learn more about this interesting but very practical approach."

Hazel Howell, Speech and Language Therapist

"GLP can be daunting and seem complex. This book is so practical, with easy to understand examples that help everyone to understand the stages of NLA. The section of scoring was especially helpful: it allows us to gain an accurate sample for scoring and setting goals for practice."

Karen Royle, Speech and Language Therapist

"This is a generous, well-researched and highly accessible resource. As well as providing background information, further reading recommendations and useful handouts, it contains clear and user-friendly advice on how to deliver interventions; from how to take case histories, to assessment, to monitoring and measuring progress, with a firm emphasis throughout on the importance of taking a person-centred approach."

Juliette Goodman, Speech and Language Therapist

Access your Online Resources

Gestalt Language Processing is accompanied by a number of printable online materials, designed to ensure this resource best supports your professional needs.

Go to https://resourcecentre.routledge.com/speechmark and click on the cover of this book.

Answer the question prompt using your copy of the book to gain access to the online content.

Gestalt Language Processing

This book invites the reader to explore Natural Language Acquisition for Gestalt Language Processors. It clearly sets out the stages of Gestalt Language Processing and the steps in therapy to effectively help neurodivergent children and young people to move on with their language development, supporting them to become independent and creative language users.

A wealth of real-life examples and in-depth case studies brings theory to life and allow practitioners to apply the principles to the children they know. Chapters include:

- A detailed description of each stage of Natural Language Acquisition and a summary of the research background.

- Clear and comprehensive guides to scoring language samples and tracking progress.

- AAC (Augmentative and Alternative Communication) options and supports for developing literacy.

- Consideration of regulation and movement supports.

- Handouts for use in practice, with extra content available online.

Gestalt Language Processing is an invaluable resource for any Speech and Language Therapist, parent or teacher who is looking to further their knowledge and transform the language support they offer to autistic and neurodivergent children.

Alison Battye is a Speech and Language Therapist with 25 years of experience supporting autistic and neurodivergent children. She is the author of three previous highly respected books on AAC and self-care for Allied Health Professionals. Ali regularly supervises other SLTs, provides training and attends speaking events to further awareness of AAC and language development for autistic and neurodivergent children.

Gestalt Language Processing

Supporting Autistic and Neurodivergent Children with Natural Language Acquisition

Alison Battye

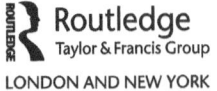

Routledge
Taylor & Francis Group

LONDON AND NEW YORK

Designed cover image: © Getty Images

First published 2025
by Routledge
4 Park Square, Milton Park, Abingdon, Oxon OX14 4RN

and by Routledge
605 Third Avenue, New York, NY 10158

Routledge is an imprint of the Taylor & Francis Group, an informa business

British Library Cataloguing-in-Publication Data
A catalogue record for this book is available from the British Library

ISBN: 978-1-032-71700-5 (hbk)
ISBN: 978-1-032-71699-2 (pbk)
ISBN: 978-1-032-71702-9 (ebk)

DOI: 10.4324/9781032717029

Typeset in Meta
by Apex CoVantage, LLC

Access the Support Material: https://resourcecentre.routledge.com/speechmark

Contents

Contents

Contents

13 GLP and literacy 191

16 Recommended reading

Contents

With heartfelt thanks to

All the GLP children I have ever worked with. You teach me so much about joy, engagement, play, the beauty of language in all its forms, and the power of multi-modal communication.

The parents and carers of the GLP children I work with. You have trusted me with your most precious people, and have allowed me to partner with you through this journey of discovery. You knew this stuff all along, and I am so sorry that it took us, as Speech and Language Therapists, so long to join you in believing in your child.

Those parents who read chapters of the book from a parent's perspective, and were incredibly supportive.

Ann Peters, Barry Prizant and Marge Blanc, for their longitudinal research, their analysis and writings, and most importantly their belief that Gestalt Language Processing was every bit as natural and communicative as Analytic Language Processing.

Marge Blanc, who generously gave up her time to discuss this project, and for providing us with the protocol of Natural Language Acquisition. Discovering this has been transformational for so many of us.

Laura Lee and Northwestern University Press for permission to reproduce the DST and DSS.

Julie Holmes and Kate Cummings, who show such inclusive leadership in the UK Natural Language Acquisition study group. Cathy Shilling who has tirelessly organised the UK GLP Conferences. It is so important that each community makes this their own, and assimilates it into our existing resources.

My peer group supervision group: Pam Hunt, Sarah Hooper and Sally Rigden. The SLTs that I supervise, and the ASLTIP book discussion group who generously read and reviewed this book. Your insights, experiences, ideas, doubts and questions have been invaluable. We all need a safe place to explore our insecurities, test our half-baked ideas, ask silly questions, be ourselves, inspire one another, and celebrate our joyful practice.

With special thanks to my longstanding speech therapy colleagues and friends, Sonia Sivyer, Wendy Callaghan, Clare Dentten, Sally Luffrum, Caroline Mitchell and Juliette Goodman. I so appreciate the love and encouragement you unfailingly provide.

And finally, my family. Stephen, my husband, for all those cups of tea and your constant calm presence. My daughters, Caty and Amelie, for believing in me, and coaching me when I was doubtful. My parents, Jan and Phil, for instilling bravery in me and being beside me every step of the way.

Chapter 1

An introduction to Gestalt Language Processing

Gestalt Language Processing (GLP) is arguably the biggest thing to happen in the world of Speech and Language Therapy in the last 20 years. Never has an approach gained so much traction and been talked about by so many, or caused such profound change in clinical pathways and advice for parents and teachers.

If you are an autistic person or a parent of an autistic child then you may not have been quite so surprised to hear that echolalia is meaningful, and that whole phrases, songs or scripts are the GLP's entry into language development.

But let's assume for the moment that we are starting from scratch. If you are a Speech and Language Therapist new to GLP you might be asking questions like:

- Does Gestalt Language Processing explain why some autistic children have been unable to benefit from our traditional advice?

- Have we been underestimating the language potential of autistic children because we did not understand their processing style?

- How does this fit in with other child-led approaches like Intensive Interaction, VERVE and Hanen?

- Can we better support non-speaking or minimally speaking children to develop and access speech?

- Is this the end of PECS and compliance-based approaches?

- What does it mean for AAC design?

- What does this mean for literacy teaching?

If these are the questions you are asking, then you are in the right place.

Right from the start I want to make it clear that I am still learning about Gestalt Language Processing. Just as with neurodiversity more generally, knowledge in this area will continue to evolve.

DOI: 10.4324/9781032717029-1

When I first started to learn about Gestalt Language Processing it very much resonated with my clinical experience and I needed to know more. My experiments with incorporating this approach have had a profound effect on me as a therapist and the children and parents that I work with. I believe it to be an approach of significant value, and I'd like to share some of my experiences. I also believe that you are an equal partner in this inquiry and will add your own insights to the mix.

A book is a snapshot in time. Inevitably, my thinking will evolve, just as yours will. This book is not intended as a static manual of steps we must take. Rather it is an invitation to explore. We all have a wealth of experience, expertise and creativity; we will approach things differently, and authentically, as individuals. We will learn from every child, parent and professional that we engage with. I hope that we continue to ask curious questions, learn from our mistakes, and grow supportive and nurturing communities.

Gestalt Language Processing and autism

Gestalt Language Processing is associated with autism but is not exclusive to autism. It is possible for someone to be a GLP and not autistic, and it is possible to be autistic and not be a GLP. But there does seem to be an overlap between autism and GLP. GLP may be associated with other neurodivergencies, e.g. ADHD, dyspraxia, dyslexia, but we just don't know precise figures at the moment.

Analytic Language Processing

In order to explain Gestalt Language Processing, it is helpful to first explain Analytic Language Processing (ALP). This is a model of language acquisition that we are familiar with. A baby moves through predictable patterns of babbling, and then one day manages to isolate a protoword, like 'dada'. The child's audience is delighted and reinforces this word and helps the child to recognise that the 'word' refers to a particular person or thing. The child starts to acquire more single words, and when they have about 50 single words in their repertoire, they start to use these words in word + word combinations like 'mummy sock', 'mummy gone' and so on. Three-word phrases follow, and so on.

This pathway relies upon the child being able to isolate single words from the continuous melodic speech sound-stream. An ALP child recognises that a word is a referential unit of meaning. The word represents a thing or person or place (noun), an action (verb), an attribute (adjective) or a position (preposition). ALPs have been described as 'word babies'.

Gestalt Language Processing

Some children might be particularly attuned to the musicality of language. Their first 'unit of meaning', to use Ann Peters' term (more on this shortly), is a melodic pattern, a sound-stream which could be a phrase, a song, a line from a story or a script from a tv programme or film. This sound-stream is the soundtrack that accompanied a meaningful experience.

These children are natural 'gestalt' processors. They can take in the 'whole experience'. This may include their location and positioning, movement patterns, sensory experiences and associated emotions. These children tend to have an excellent memory for whole experiences. They recall whole episodes in detail, and are described as having superior 'episodic' memory.

These children's first attempts at speech are long unintelligible strings. They reproduce the 'tune' to a phrase, with its intonation pattern. These children are not yet recognising individual words within the sound-stream. Their early forays into language might sound like 'awuva teye mooyanba'. Much later on, when the child's speech motor skills have developed, this phrase may sound much more like 'I love you to the moon and back'.

Because GLPs tune into the suprasegmental aspects of speech first (the tune and rhythm), they have been described as 'intonation babies'.

The following figure offers a visual description of how analytic language development and gestalt language development differ.

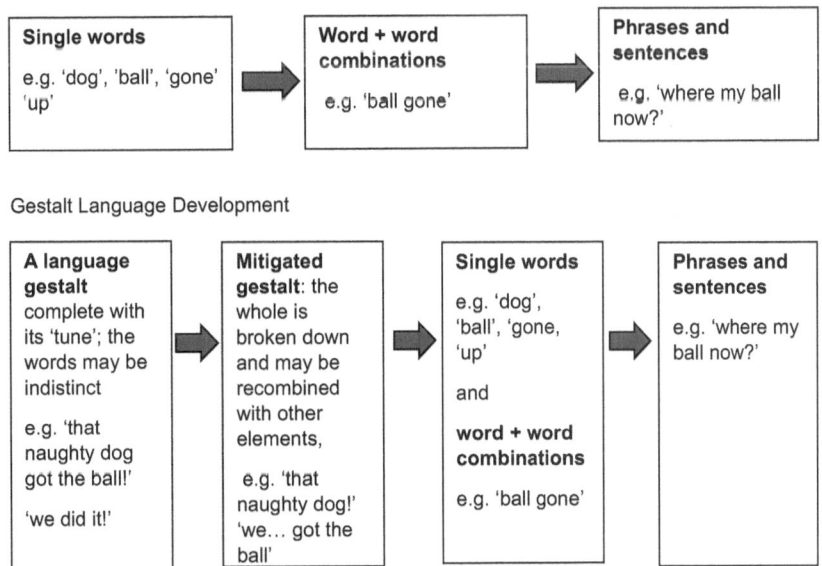

Single words	Word + word combinations	Phrases and sentences
e.g. 'dog', 'ball', 'gone' 'up'	e.g. 'ball gone'	e.g. 'where my ball now?'

Gestalt Language Development

A language gestalt complete with its 'tune'; the words may be indistinct	Mitigated gestalt: the whole is broken down and may be recombined with other elements,	Single words	Phrases and sentences
e.g. 'that naughty dog got the ball!' 'we did it!'	e.g. 'that naughty dog!' 'we... got the ball'	e.g. 'dog', 'ball', 'gone, 'up' and word + word combinations e.g. 'ball gone'	e.g. 'where my ball now?'

It is important to note that these models describe extremes at either end of a continuum. It is likely that we all fall along this continuum and use both strategies to some extent.

Figure 1.1 A comparison of analytic versus gestalt language development

A gestalt is more than the sum of its parts

A dictionary definition of gestalt is:

> *something such as a structure or experience that, when considered as a whole, has qualities that are more than the total of all its parts*

A gestalt is the whole experience. It might include the details of the room or location, and the exact positions of people or objects. It might include actions and bodily sensations. It might include sensory experiences: the quality of light, the sensation of touch, a smell, a taste. It is very likely to include the emotional resonance of the experience. And importantly, for language acquisition, it may include the soundtrack to that experience: what someone said, including their voice quality, tone of voice, volume, intonation pattern and the feeling behind it. This could also be a song, a line from a story, even a whole tv programme or movie.

Because GLPs retain aspects of an experience that ALPs have likely forgotten, they can make profound and creative connections between past experiences and the current situation. Because of the emotional resonance aspect of a gestalt, GLPs are often able to convey an extremely nuanced message, which gets to the heart of the matter.

Take 5-year-old Alex. When his mum completed an impressive driving manoeuvre, he used a line from *Wreck-It Ralph:* 'you are one *dynamite gal*'. Or 4-year-old Aria, who, when she is uninterested in an activity says with a sigh: 'it was a dreary day for all of the animals'.

We have probably all had this experience from the line of a song or poem, or a favourite movie quote, where it perfectly fits with our experience. We are moved beyond the simple meaning of the words. There is something more: emotional resonance, shared experience, humour, pathos, connection with the human condition. A gestalt is more than the sum of its parts.

Sometimes a child's language gestalts are a little more obscure, and we will need to do some detective work to infer a child's communication intentions. Take Aria again. She uses the phrase 'Hammer time!' when she doesn't want an adult to touch her toys. Aria's mum was able to explain to me that this comes from the MC Hammer song, *You can't touch this*!

Another child, 4-year-old Azariah, says, 'seven!' when he is distressed. We haven't been able to identify the origin of this gestalt, but the communication intention is clear from the contexts in which he uses it. In fact, we can never know the exact meaning of a language gestalt: it is so individual for that child. But we can infer, and respond accordingly.

A natural Gestalt Language Processor will likely always be drawn to gestalt communication, and we do not want to change this. This approach is about honouring the natural tendencies of an individual, building trust so that the individual can share this world of communication, and creating conditions whereby further language options are available.

Language acquisition research

Back in the 1970s and 1980s, there were many longitudinal studies of how children naturally acquired language. Researchers including Roger Brown,[1] Lois Bloom[2] and Katherine Nelson[3] focused on the semantic-syntactic structures that children learnt and what sequence. They concluded that there was a predictable pattern where the mean length of utterance (MLU) gradually became longer and longer, from single words to two-word combinations and so on.

Ruth Clark[4] noticed that not all children used the same strategies, noting that

> **One boy seemed to have strategies for simplifying the tasks of speech reception and production. He would incorporate the immediately prior utterance, or some portion of it, intact into his utterance as if to avoid structuring his entire utterance from scratch. Another strategy was to extend his repertoire of structures to express more complex ideas simply by combining two existing structures without reordering any of the elements to match adult syntax.**

In her research papers[5] and subsequent book *The Units of Language Acquisition*,[6] Ann Peters used the term 'gestalt' to describe a pattern of language acquisition that she observed in her research in the 1970s. She observed that whilst some children acquired predominantly single words as the first 'units of language acquisition', other children often acquired whole phrases. These phrases were difficult to transcribe, because the child's speech motor system was at this stage unable to cope with such complex sound patterns. Such long streams of babble-like utterances, possibly containing a recognisable word or two, were also difficult for researchers to attribute meaning to. A parent could make a good guess, because they might recognise a chunk of language from a song or rhyme, from a favourite play routine or an episode of life. This was the first indication that we need to partner with parents in order to truly understand language acquisition!

'Frame-and-slot' model

Peters referenced the work of other linguistics researchers who noted this tendency for children to acquire chunks of language as well as single words (Bloom 1970,[7] Bloom 1975,[8] Clark 1974,[9] Nagy 1978,[10] MacWhinney 1978[11]). There was a recognition that in addition to a lexicon of single words, we also learn language by storing prefabricated chunks of language. These chunks might be used wholesale or 'remixed' later.

In many ways this is an efficient way to learn language, and this strategy is often seen in sequential second language acquisition. There is a natural progression from the acquisition of the original gestalt (the unanalysed whole) whereby the gestalt is broken down (or mitigated) to create a 'frame-and-slot' model for new utterances.

Now separate chunks can be slotted together to form new utterances. For instance:

Let's   *jump!*
                go
                do it again

We need   *more*
                our shoes
                this one

Ann Peters suggested that children may apply both strategies: single word learning, and also whole phrase learning, when acquiring language. Certain children may have a preference for one strategy over another, and so may be termed predominantly analytic (single word route) or predominantly gestalt (whole phrase route). It is also possible that some children are naturally 'dual processors', comfortable from the start with both strategies.

It is important to note that the 'frame-and-slot' model has been researched extensively[12–17] and has not been lost to history. It is just that the terms 'Gestalt Language Processing' and 'Analytic Language Processing' were not used by researchers in child language acquisition, and so did not pop up in literature review (until very recently).

Why has ALP dominated our profession?

Peters identified that the gestalt pathway may have been overlooked in the research because gestalts are so difficult to transcribe and attribute meaning to. The research that we have relied on in the field of Speech and Language Therapy (e.g. Bloom 1973,[18] Brown 1973[19]) may inadvertently have been missing data, because unclear gestalts were not included in the language analysis. Other research did reference the role of prefabricated chunks of language, or the 'frame-and-slot' model (Clark 1974,[20] Nelson 1981[21]), but this has not informed speech and language interventions so much as analytical strategies.

Do we all use both analytic and gestalt strategies?

Peters observed that Minh, the first Gestalt Language Processor that she studied,[22] used gestalt strategies for some language functions and analytic strategies for others. Minh used gestalt strategies for opening conversations ('what's that?' 'uh-oh!'), in play routines ('aeroplane go up!'), requesting ('I want milk'), commenting ('silly, isn't it?') and reproducing a phrase from a book. He used analytic strategies for labelling pictures in a book ('horsie', 'doggie'), labelling a quality ('hot', 'cool') and requesting an object or action ('cookie', 'milk', 'up').

It is possible that whilst analytic strategies resonate with some children, and gestalt strategies resonate with others, there is a continuum between. Being at one end of the gestalt continuum could account for the limited response we see from some autistic children to a purely analytic approach.

The role of echolalia

Following the language acquisition research in the 1970s, a slightly different but related research route was taken up in the 1980s by Barry Prizant[23,24] who observed that 'language patterns such as immediate and delayed echolalia . . . can be better understood as manifestations of gestalt processing'.[25]

One of Prizant's vital contributions was that echolalia is not mere parroting, devoid of communicative intent.[26] His research showed that both immediate and delayed echolalia served a range of communication functions.

Immediate echolalia, or speech that is immediately echoed back, could be used communicatively to:

- Maintain the interaction and take a turn.

- Label an object or action.

- Affirm a prior utterance.

- Request an object or action.

And also non-communicatively to:

- Signal dysregulation or pain.

- Accompany a regulating activity.

- Be used as a rehearsal strategy.

Delayed echolalia, or speech that is repeated later, was used communicatively to:

- Complete familiar verbal routines.

- Provide new information.

- Protest.

- Gain attention.

- Direct another person's actions.

And non-communicatively to:

- Draw a connection with a previous experience.

- Practice language skills.

- Self-regulate.

Prizant went on to describe gestalt language acquisition in autistic children whereby they started with echolalia, with whole phrases or language chunks (gestalts). These were then broken down into smaller chunks, and then the chunks could be recombined and co-joined. He termed these changed phrases 'mitigated echolalia' or 'mitigations'. There was then further breaking down of the language chunks into single words. Only once this process had begun could novel 'from scratch', self-generated phrases and sentences begin.[27]

These four stages of language acquisition were soon to be tested and expanded upon by Marge Blanc.

Natural Language Acquisition (NLA)

Marge Blanc's longitudinal studies of language acquisition of autistic children were reported in a series of articles[28] and then in her book *Natural Language Acquisition on the Autism Spectrum.*[29] Blanc described Gestalt Language Processors as children who naturally:

- Acquire whole phrases rather than single words in their early language development.

- Have a musical quality to their speech, being described as richly intonational.

- Pick up whole rhymes, songs and scripts.

- Use these phrases or scripts to make connections between experiences.

- Have a preference for language that is emotionally resonant.

Blanc described six stages of gestalt language acquisition. These stages are shown in Table 1.1 adapted from Blanc et al (2023)[30]:

Table 1.1 The six stages of Natural Language Acquisition

		Examples
Stage 1	Language gestalts (wholes, scripts, songs, language soundtracks from experiences)	Zoom zoom zoom, we're going to the moon! It's a dinosaur!
Stage 2	Mitigations: a) Shortening long gestalts b) Dividing them into chunks c) Recombining different chunks	We're going to the moon! We're going! We're going to the shops! It's an octopus!
Stage 3	Isolated single words Word + word combinations of referential single words	dinosaur; rocket dinosaur . . . big; rocket . . . up
Stage 4	Original phrases and beginning sentences	We got dinosaur Put rocket up there
Stage 5	Original sentences with more complex grammar	I can get the dinosaurs I don't want to put my shoes on
Stage 6	Original sentences culminating in a complete grammar system	Who could have taken the dinosaurs? I've been looking for my shoes

Now it is fair to say that Blanc's research was based on a relatively small number of children and that these children were very clearly GLP. We may see children like this, and also children who use both GLP and ALP strategies, as well as children who are predominantly ALPs.

Children will nearly always have language from different stages, and the stages overlap. I see this as a production line, with language coming in at stage 1 and being processed through stage 2 mitigations, and so on. Gradually a child's language spreads through the stages so that more of their language is made up of later stages. It is possible that once a child has moved through stage 3, they no longer need new language to enter at stage 1, but can process new vocabulary at stage 3 and use it immediately in original sentences. Each child is unique because brains are unique. This process can take months or years, and it is difficult to predict progress, but progress within each stage is profound, offering more variety of language and flexibility of language use.

Why are we hearing so much about GLP now?

The interest in Gestalt Language Processing has accompanied a wider cultural shift towards recognising and celebrating neurodiversity. Our culture has been dominated by the neurotypical majority, and neurominorities have been sidelined. Many autistic adults now have a voice on social media and in public speaking platforms, and have written their own accounts of what it is like to live in a society that advantages neurotypicals.

Barry Prizant and Marge Blanc were early advocates for autistic people. With the influence of social media and a global pandemic perhaps facilitating online collaboration, awareness of this work has grown. Alexandria Zachos, a practising Speech Language Pathologist in the US, has been incredibly successful in spreading awareness through social media and online training. Blanc's work has resonated with thousands of parents and Speech and Language Therapists globally, who are now taking up the baton with their own longitudinal research with multilingual children, older students, AAC users and so on.

Future research

This work will continue to evolve: every child's pathway is unique, and can add to our understanding and appreciation of Natural Language Acquisition (Figure 1.2).

The NLA approach uses language sampling to collect data. With language sampling, there is potentially a wealth of longitudinal data that might be studied in more detail. With modern recording methods using smart phones, and techniques such

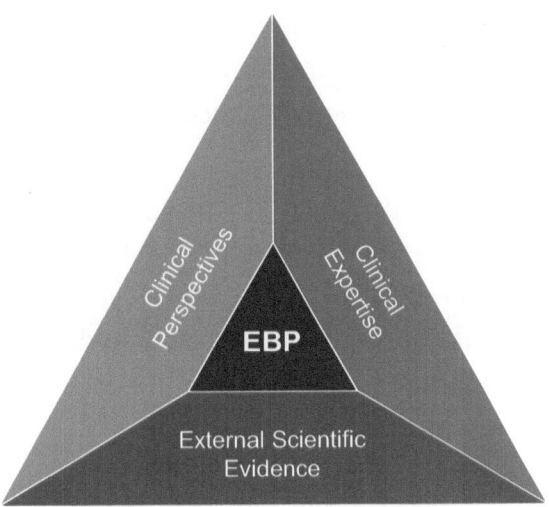

Figure 1.2 The evidence-based practice triangle

as 'traceback', this process of data collection is likely to become easier to analyse. Perhaps a future application of Artificial Intelligence (AI) might help this process to become more efficient.

This is very much a 'grass-roots' movement which includes parents and autistic people at its core. Bilingual and multilingual populations are integral in current research. Every GLP child is adding to our understanding of this evolving framework.

Our professional bodies require the use of evidence-based practice. In recent years our profession has perhaps been overly concerned with one side of the evidence-based practice triangle, the 'external scientific evidence', at the expense of 'clinical expertise' and, crucially, 'client perspectives'. It is easier to gather 'data' in discrete trials where a child has to repeat the same very limited behaviour in a highly controlled situation. This has led to interventions which autistic and neurodivergent people are telling us have taught them to mask their neurodivergence. This has caused them harm, impacting on their sense of self and their trust in communication partners. Their experience of therapy has been traumatic. Therapists too have felt a misalignment between their core values and what they have been trained to do. They have felt uncomfortable breaching bodily autonomy (using hand-over-hand), instructing a child how to communicate and withholding items until a child requests them in the correct manner. It is time to reconsider this. We need to rebalance the triangle.

Clinical implications

In many ways, this is not an 'intervention'. The term Natural Language Acquisition implies that under the right circumstances this process happens *naturally*. We can partner with parents in order to nurture the right conditions for GLP to flourish. It may be that only a portion of GLP children need regular one-to-one therapy. As a profession, we need to consider universal advice, as well as specialist advice.

Where intervention *is* needed, Speech and Language Therapists can join children and parents in a partnership to explore how the NLA framework might help to support a child. Whilst weekly play-based therapy may be optimal for some children, others may benefit from a parent coaching model. Training for educators is an urgent need, to allow appropriate language modelling throughout the day.

With neurodiversity awareness and advocacy, we are recognising the importance of client perspectives in assessing our therapeutic interventions. NLA describes six stages of language acquisition, but it is not the aim that everyone should be aiming for the same outcome. We need to honour the natural language of autistic individuals, and for many, they may choose the joy of gestalts and mitigations of stages1 and 2. Stage 1 gestalts have a richly resonant quality which can never be matched by analytic language. Stage 2 mitigations can be incredibly flexible and wide-ranging. NLA describes the stages but does not prescribe them. This approach honours the communication choices of the individual.

A note on terminology

I use the term 'GLP' as shorthand for 'a child who predominantly uses gestalt strategies to acquire language'. It is likely that we are all somewhere on a continuum between being extreme Gestalt Language Processors and extreme analytic processors. Children who largely use echolalia and show other clear signs of gestalt processing are towards the extreme gestalt end. Those children who use a mix of gestalt and analytic strategies are unlikely to need SLT intervention, but if they do, then using the strategies in this book is likely to be helpful. Therapists may also experiment with supporting them with more traditional ALP strategies in addition. We use our clinical judgement to assess what is working for an individual child.

I use identity-first language rather than person-first language. That is, I say 'autistic child', rather than 'child with autism'. This is because the majority of autistic adults prefer this. Autism is a vital and valued part of their identity, and not a medical condition which needs to be fixed.

For ease of reading, I tend to use 'child' rather than 'child or young person'. I made this difficult editorial decision just because sometimes as a writer you have to choose one path and be consistent. For those of you who find this choice irksome, I sincerely apologise.

I use the term 'non-speaking' rather than non-verbal. Non-verbal implies that a person does not understand language, and this is not the case with the vast majority of non-speaking people. It is just the physical act of speaking that is inaccessible.

A significant proportion of autistic adults experience times when their speech is inaccessible, and so they use AAC. They have times when they use 'mouth words' and times when they use their AAC words. I have used the term 'part-time AAC user' to describe this.

I am working towards eliminating deficit-based language from my practice and my writing. I aim to celebrate and honour neurodivergent experiences, but there are inevitably limitations to my perspective. Please bear with me whilst I learn.

Notes

1 Brown, R. (1973) *A First Language: The Early Stages* Cambridge, MA: Harvard University Press.
2 Bloom, L. (1970) *Language Development: Form and Function in Emerging Grammars* Cambridge, MA: MIT Press; Bloom, L., Lightbown, P. & Hood, L. (1975) 'Structure and variation in child language' *Monographs of the Society for Research in Child Development* 40(2, Serial No. 160).
3 Nelson, K. (1973) 'Structure and strategy in learning to talk' *Monographs of the Society for Research in Child Development* 38(1–2, Serial No 149), 136.
4 Clark, R. (1974) 'Performing without competence' *Journal of Child Language* 1(1), 1–10.
5 Peters, A. (1977) 'Language learning strategies: Does the whole equal the sum of the parts?' *Language* 53(3), 560–573.
6 Peters, A. (1983) *The Units of Language Acquisition* Cambridge University Press.
7 Bloom, L. (1970) *Language Development: Form and Function in Emerging Grammars* Cambridge, MA: MIT Press.
8 Bloom, L., Lightbown, P. & Hood, L. (1975) 'Structure and variation in child language' *Monographs of the Society for Research in Child Development* 40(2, Serial No. 160).
9 Clark, R. (1974) 'Performing without competence' *Journal of Child Language* 1(1), 1–10.
10 Nagy, W. (1978) 'Some non-idiom larger-than-word units in the lexicon' *Papers from the Parasession on the Lexicon' Chicago Linguistic Society*, 289–300.
11 MacWhinney, B. (1978) 'The acquisition of morphophonology' *Monographs of the Society for Research in Child Development* 43(1–2, Serial No. 174).

12 Tomasello, M. (2000) 'First steps toward a usage-based theory of language acquisition' *Cognitive Linguistics* 11(1/2), 61–82.

13 Tomasello, M. (2003) *Constructing a Language: A Usage-Based Theory of Language Acquisition* Cambridge, MA: Harvard University Press.

14 Lieven, E., Behrens, H., Speares, J. & Tomasello, M. (2003) 'Early syntactic creativity: A usage-based approach' *Journal of Child Language* 30, 333–370.

15 Dąbrowska, E. (2004) 'Recycling utterances: A speaker's guide to sentence processing' *Cognitive Linguistics* 25(4), 615–653.

16 Dąbrowska, E. & Lieven, E. (2005) 'Towards a lexically specific grammar of children's question constructions' *Cognitive Linguistics* 16(3), 437–474.

17 Lieven, E., Salomo, D. & Tomasello, M. (2009) 'Two-year-old children's production of multi-word utterances: A usage-based analysis' *Cognitive Linguistics* 20, 481–507.

18 Bloom, L. (1973) *One Word at a Time* The Hague: Mouton.

19 Brown, R. (1973) *A First Language: The Early Stages* Cambridge, MA: Harvard University Press.

20 Clark, R. (1974) 'Performing without competence' *Journal of Child Language* 1, 1–10.

21 Nelson, K. (1981) 'Individual differences in language development: Implications for development and language' *Developmental Psychology* 17, 170–187.

22 Peters, A. (1977) 'Language learning strategies: Does the whole equal the sum of the parts?' *Language* 53(3).

23 Prizant, B. & Duchan, J. (1981) 'The functions of immediate echolalia in autistic children' *Journal of Speech and Hearing Disorders* 46, 241–249.

24 Prizant, B. (1982) 'Gestalt language and gestalt processing in autism' *Topics in Language Disorders* 3(1), 16–23.

25 Prizant, B. (1983) 'Language acquisition and communicative behavior in autism: Toward an understanding of the "whole" of it' *Journal of Speech and Hearing Disorders* 48, 296–307.

26 Prizant, B. & Rydell, P. (1984) 'Analysis of functions of delayed echolalia in autistic children' *Journal of Speech and Hearing Research* 27, 183–192.

27 Prizant, B. M. & Rydell, P. J. (1993) 'Assessment and intervention considerations for unconventional verbal behavior' *Communicative Alternatives to Challenging Behavior: Integrating Functional Assessment and Intervention Strategies* 3, 263–297.

28 Blanc, M. (2005) 'Finding the words to tell the "whole" story: Natural Language Acquisition on the Autistic Spectrum' *Autism and Asperger's Digest*, May–June, July–August, September–October, November–December; Blanc, M. (2006) 'Finding the words . . . when it's hard to find your voice' *Autism and Asperger's Digest*, January–February, March–April; Blanc, M. (2006) 'Finding the words . . . when they are pictures' *Autism and Asperger's Digest*, May–June, July–August, September–October, November–December; Blanc, M. (2007) 'Finding the words . . . when they are in there somewhere' *Autism and Asperger's Digest*, January–February, March–April, May–June, July–August; Blanc, M. (2008 and 2009) 'Finding the words . . . with augmented communication' *Autism and Asperger's Digest*, May–June, July–August, September–October, November–December,

January–February; Blanc, M. (2009) 'Finding the words . . . to self-regulate' *Autism Digest*, March–April, May–June, July–August, September–October, November–December.

29 Blanc, M. (2012) *Natural Language Acquisition on the Autism Spectrum: The Journey from Echolalia to Self-Generated Language* Madison, WI: Communication Development Center, Inc.

30 Blanc, M., Blackwell, A. & Elias, P. (2023) 'Using the natural language acquisition protocol to support Gestalt language development' *Perspectives of the ASHA Special Interest Groups*.

Chapter 2

Identification and partnership

Gestalt Language Processing is a manifestation of gestalt cognitive processing

As Barry Prizant taught us, Gestalt Language Processing is a manifestation of wider, more general, gestalt processing. There will be clues that a child thinks in whole experiences through their play and everyday routines. They might recall episodes of life with much richer detail than analytic processors. They are likely to surprise those around them with their recall of episodes that others have forgotten. For example, when they pass a layby where the family's car broke down three years ago, they will do or say something to indicate that they remember this. They might remember that they ate mints whilst they waited for the pickup truck to arrive, or that there was a blown-out tyre by the side of the road.

Gestalt processing might be revealed in the child's assumptions about what is going to happen if a situation is repeated. For example, if they go to the doctors' they may sit in the same chair and lift their top up because last time the doctor examined their chest.

A gestalt processor is likely to have a preference for completing one experience before transitioning to the next. Interrupting this process is likely to be as distressing or annoying as an unfinished line in a favourite song, or removing a last piece of a puzzle so that it can't be completed.

A gestalt processor may not like sets of items to be split up: the alphabet is a perfect whole, numbers from one to ten are a perfect whole, a rainbow arrangement of pencils is a perfect whole. Splitting up these sets is the equivalent of us ripping the arm off a favourite teddy. We must rid ourselves of the notion that these children are being 'rigid' and 'inflexible': our demands for them to break their gestalt at this stage are unreasonable.

Signs of Gestalt Language Processing

A good indicator that a child is a GLP is that they are not following the analytic language acquisition pathway. They may have acquired some single words, but these do not then become word + word combinations. If their first natural first step in language acquisition is to have the 'whole' and then break down the whole,

DOI: 10.4324/9781032717029-2

a single word does not give them any scope for progression. A longer chunk of language would be more helpful.

Other signs include:

- The child uses long strings of babble-like utterances, often unintelligible, perhaps with one or two recognisable words within them.

- The child marks the number of syllables in a phrase, but the words are not clear.

- The utterances follow distinct intonational patterns. The phrase is said with the same intonation pattern each time.

- The utterance may include certain body movements or gestures, e.g. spreading arms out wide, jumping.

- There may be a distinct voice quality or an accent, which has been retained from the original sound source.

- The child responds positively to music, songs and rhymes, more so than single words in shared play routines.

- The child likes watching, rewinding and rewatching the same video clips on YouTube or other media sources.

- The child seems to be quoting dialogue from video clips, tv or film. Again the individual words are unclear, but the intonation pattern is there.

- The child seems to particularly love phrases that are rich in emotional meaning. They will be spoken emphatically to convey strong emotions.

- The child may use a gestalt phrase to make an association between a past experience and what is happening now. There is something about the current situation that reminds them of when they first heard their phrase.

- The child echoes back what has been said so that they would use a 'you' pronoun instead of an 'I' pronoun, e.g. 'do you want milk?' when they mean 'I want milk'.

- The child may be highly unintelligible, only using open vocalisations with no consonants. They may hum the tune of songs, scripts, phrases or words.

- A non-speaking child may reveal their gestalt tendencies by showing gestalt cognitive processing: they may act out gestalts through body movements, or expect a particular experience to unfold in exactly the same way each time, including extraneous parts that were only present in their first experience.

- The child might love sets of items, e.g. the whole alphabet, all the pieces of a puzzle or components of a building set. They do not like these being broken up or disrupted by adult suggestions (at least in stage 1. In stage 2, this begins to be more acceptable).

- The child likes to complete a routine or a task, and does not like being interrupted mid-flow. Again this is likely to become more flexible as they move through NLA stages.

- The child needs structure and predictability in their routines.

- At an earlier stage in development, they used echolalia, but have since become minimally or non-speaking. They may whisper their gestalts, use only character voices, or even have internalised this language, and it is now not possible for us to hear it.

- The child has not responded to traditional SLT advice. The copy-and-add strategy of copying back what they have said and adding a word does not seem to work for them.

Parents will generally be able to identify if their child is a GLP. Once we list a few of these indications, the parent may give us examples that they have noted themselves. They will likely have been supporting their child's language development very naturally by following their train of thought. They know their child so well that they can identify where a phrase or an intonation pattern has come from, and what it means for a child.

Language gestalts are not literal

A GLP's stage 1 language will not be literal. There will be some phrases that are close to literal: 'up you come!' as they climb the stairs, 'whoopsadaisy!' when they drop something. But there will likely be less literal phrases that only those close to the child can easily understand. For example, the child sings 'I can sing a rainbow' when they are sad. They do this because their granny comforted them with this song when they hurt themselves. The gestalt phrase is the soundtrack from the original experience which has an emotional resonance relevant to the current situation.

It is perfectly acceptable to have a working hypothesis that a child is a GLP and begin modelling language accordingly. If they respond to this approach with engagement and enjoyment, we have evidence that they are a GLP.

What are the six stages of Natural Language Acquisition?

In Table 2.1 are the six stages of GLP Natural Language Acquisition, which we will return to in later chapters. It is only by getting to know a child well that we can start to understand where they are in their GLP language acquisition.

Table 2.1 The six stages of Natural Language Acquisition

		Examples
Stage 1	Language gestalts (wholes, scripts, songs, language soundtracks from experiences)	Zoom zoom zoom, we're going to the moon! It's a dinosaur!
Stage 2	Mitigations: a) Shortening long gestalts b) Dividing them into chunks c) Recombining different chunks	We're going to the moon! We're going! We're going to the shops! It's an octopus!
Stage 3	Isolated single words Word + word combinations of referential single words	dinosaur; rocket dinosaur . . . big; rocket . . . up
Stage 4	Original phrases and beginning sentences	We got dinosaur Put rocket up there
Stage 5	Original sentences with more complex grammar	I can get the dinosaurs I don't want to put my shoes on
Stage 6	Original sentences culminating in a complete grammar system	Who could have taken the dinosaurs? I've been looking for my shoes

We will always see several stages coexisting at any one time. I see this as a production line: new language comes in at stage 1, and is then processed through subsequent stages. A child who has a lot of stage 4 language will still acquire stage 1 gestalts. These new gestalts may later be broken down and recombined, and release new words that can move through stage 3, 4 and beyond. This production line gets more efficient as a child moves through the stages. In stage 4 and beyond, the production line process may happen immediately, or internally.

It is not in every child's future to acquire full stage 6 language. For all children it will make a huge difference for the adults around them to understand the communication intentions behind their stage 1 gestalts. This will allow connection and communication to flourish. They will then likely go on to break down these gestalts and recombine chunks to create new, more flexible phrases. This opens opportunities for communicating with many more people in many different contexts. A stage 2 communicator is seen by society as more competent, and so they are given many more opportunities to interact and practice their language skills.

It is desirable that a child moves through all the stages, and can ultimately acquire stage 6 academic language. Children who are identified and supported at a young age as GLPs may move through the stages relatively quickly.

What about older GLPs?

GLP children who have not been correctly identified and who have had only analytic strategies for language modelling may have gotten stuck at stage 1. Stage 1 gestalts can include single words, and taught phrases like 'I want a biscuit'.

When a child has a lot of stuck single word gestalts, there is nowhere for them to go with them. Their single word gestalts may be full of rich meanings, or telling a whole story about that entity. The word 'ice-cream' may mean 'remember when we went to the park and I had that delicious ice-cream?' If the word is not being combined in any other ways, it is likely a stuck gestalt. A phrase like 'it's my favourite' or 'I love this!' would offer more scope for stage 2 mitigations: it can be broken down and recombined in a way that 'ice-cream' cannot.

We will need to get to know a child in order to judge whether a single word is a stage 1 gestalt, a stage 2 mitigation (trimmed down from a longer phrase) or a stage 3 referential word. If it always is said in the same way with the same intonation pattern; if it is not accompanied by pointing; if it does not appear in combination with other words, it is likely to be a gestalt.

It is also possible for a child to be stuck with single word gestalts or taught phrases with their AAC. PECS is likely to result in a very small repertoire of taught phrases like 'I want biscuit' that only results in more requests starting with the words 'I want'.

To support a child who is non-speaking or minimally speaking, their AAC also needs to provide the richness of phrases, which reflect a range of communication intentions, beyond simple requesting.

Chapter 12 will explore this in more detail and provide suggestions for AAC solutions for GLPs.

Partnering with parents and professionals

I recommend signposting families, teachers and other professionals to Marge Blanc's 'Communication Development Center' website or Alex Zachos' 'Meaningful Speech' website. In the handouts section is an 'Introduction to GLP' handout that you may also share.

A young stage 1 GLP is likely to be quite unintelligible. Saying whole phrases is more than a young child's speech development can manage. Over time they will become more intelligible, but in the early days we will need a parent's help. The parents (or siblings) are much more likely to recognise the intonational contours of a phrase from everyday life, a movie or a story, because they have lived it with their child.

It is useful for those who interact with a stage 1 GLP to have a shared document that logs the child's phrases and the likely communication intention of each. This will always be a work-in-progress. There will be some gestalts that are more obscure than others, and will take time to figure out. The shared document is a way of sharing insights and ideas. The priority is to foster connection and understanding with the child, and we need one another's help to do this. You will find a language tracker document in the handouts section of this book.

Spreading awareness of NLA and GLP

Our advice for GLPs is quite different to traditional advice. Much of the standard Speech and Language Therapy advice has involved starting with single words and teaching a few functional phrases, usually around requesting objects. There is work to be done in revising advice that we share with others.

When our existing knowledge is being questioned we are likely to resist the new information, and so this may generate some unease. It is helpful to recall how we felt when we first heard about GLP. We may have felt undermined, or insecure. We may have felt overwhelmed with the complexity of the information.

The effects of supporting a child using the NLA framework generally speak for themselves.

If a professional has had experience of working with autistic children, this information tends to click. They recognise the role of gestalts in communication.

Joyful therapy

One of the biggest impacts of NLA is that a child's current communication is recognised. We are able to see that they are communicators. A child feels our faith in them. This is powerful. When a child knows we are listening, they communicate more.

If you have not yet implemented this approach, you are in for a treat. If we are willing to follow the GLP, trust them, see the world through their eyes and experience it wholly, be our most authentic self alongside of them, then I promise that this is going to be one of the most rewarding experiences of your life.

Case study: Abbas

Abbas's mum Noor contacted me because she was looking for support for her son who she suspected was autistic. He was 3½ years old. His language had been developing along typical lines until he was about 20 months old, when he had stopped talking. Noor told me that Abbas was currently vocalising tunefully, and used one recognisable word, 'dada'.

Noor described how Abbas communicated by leading adults by the hand and pushing their hand towards a toy he wanted them to operate, or towards the object he would like. Noor said that Abbas loved rhymes and songs, and watching these on YouTube. His favourites were Cocomelon and Super Simple songs. He also loved to jump and spin. He played with cars, balls and alphabet letters.

Noor brought Abbas for his first session. Abbas loved bouncing on the trampoline, and looked and smiled when I sang 'Five little monkeys'. We played several rounds of this, with Abbas joining in with the action for 'no more monkeys bouncing on the bed'.

Abbas was repeating a sequence of sounds, made up of vowels and clicks, which Noor identified as the 'ee-ay-ee-ay-oh' in 'Old Macdonald'. I sang this song, and Abbas's face lit up. I happened to have this song on my toy record player, which Abbas discovered next. He was delighted when he recognised the tune, and was happy for me to join in and sing it too. Abbas danced to the music.

Abbas then found the xylophone toy, and first played it by banging his hand on the keys, then picking up a stick and banging the keys loudly. He went to his mum for a cuddle and she said 'I love you!' Abbas returned to the record-player. I said, 'let's do it again!' and Abbas danced whilst the music played. Abbas then went back to the xylophone, repeating the sequence of banging the keys with his hand, then the stick, then going to his mum for a cuddle, and then coming back to the record-player and taking my hand to the dial to turn it.

Abbas repeated this circuit several times in the session. This was indicating to me that he was a gestalt processor: he had learnt this sequence as a whole, and was recreating it each time.

Because we had by now established a connection, and Abbas trusted that I was going to follow his lead most of the time, he watched when I picked up another xylophone stick and ran it down the keyboard to make a nice sound. I said, 'it sounds like magic!' and Abbas looked at me. The next circuit of his play, he looked at my xylophone stick and waited for me to run it down the whole keyboard before he banged the keys with his stick. This new action was incorporated into our play sequence. It was, in essence, a play mitigation!

Noor commented that Abbas would not usually be so comfortable with a new adult, and would not play for so long. We talked about recognising and validating all of his communication, including when he looked at an object, sang a possible snippet of a song, and explored making different sounds. I suggested that Noor add a song, rhyme or a consistent phrase to actions they carried out regularly. For example, singing 'up, up, up the stairs' every time they go up the stairs, and 'this is the way we wash our hands' when they washed their hands. We talked about how we were going to provide an interesting and engaging soundtrack to accompany experiences. I suggested that Noor experiment with musical intonation when she tried out fun phrases, perhaps playing with rhythm and funny voices. I gave Noor some written information about GLP, and we booked Abbas in for weekly therapy sessions.

Chapter 3

Foundational principles

Connection comes first

We can only partner with a child in their Natural Language Acquisition if we enable connection. We have to be willing to see the world through their eyes, play in the way they prefer to play, honour their sensory and movement needs, listen deeply, use the communication modes that come naturally to them and see them as a competent communicator. We have to throw off any pretensions of being an expert, because the child is going to lead us.

Multi-modal communication may include modes we have not thought about

In Julia Bascom's anthology of autistic voices, *Loud Hands*,[1] contributors discuss how their natural language might be in communication modes that neurotypicals have not been recognising.

These modes might be:

- The way their hands or bodies move.

- The visual patterns they are exploring and sharing.

- The images they are drawn to or are making.

- The objects that they delight in . . .

These modes may not be immediately obvious to neurotypical communication partners. We will need to slow down and stop talking to be able to notice what modes the child is using, and to be open to the possible messages they are trying to convey.

- Are they arranging items in particular patterns or types of constructions?

- Are there themes in their play that they return to again and again?

- What is it about the objects that they are drawn to that delights them?

- Can we join them and gain appreciation of this mode?

- If they seek out images or text, how can we support this?

DOI: 10.4324/9781032717029-3

- Can we communicate through taking photos? Drawing? Building? Arranging? Appreciating sparkles? Pressing objects to our faces?

We have to be open to more modes of communication than we dreamt of.

The child is allowed to be their authentic self, and so are we

Children can simply be themselves with this approach. They are not needing to follow a structured programme. We are not requiring compliance, and we are not aiming for them to appear more neurotypical. Their child is allowed to be themselves, to seek out their favourite sensory and motor experiences, to immerse themselves in their interests and enthusiasms, and to share their unique perspective on the world. No one is going to try to stop their child 'stimming' or echoing language. Everything that the child says or does is presumed to be meaningful, communicative and important. Our role is simply to join them, and keep the connection going. We as therapists let go of any pretensions of being 'the therapist' with a box of tricks. We only have to 'be' with a child. This is a highly mindful approach: we are just here with the child, sharing the moment.

We partner with parents

Parents know their child. They typically know the myriad ways in which their child is communicating. They can read their child's body language. They know their interests and enthusiasms. They know many of the memorable episodes in life that gave rise to stage 1 gestalts. They can draw in siblings to help if they can't identify a particular song or movie script. They are there when the child reads or writes for the first time, or creates a picture or a scene in their play which is important. If we are working one-to-one with a child, we will need to liaise closely with a parent, because they will have the answers to many of our questions.

Strengths-based language

Parents who have been through an autism diagnosis (or diagnosis for other developmental conditions) for their child may have become accustomed to professionals talking about their child in terms of deficits. We have an opportunity and a responsibility to change this narrative into a strengths-based model.

Neurodivergent children often teach us how to be in the moment. Autistic children give us access to new sensory and motor experiences that we may have lost touch with. GLPs amaze us with their creative ways of using language, making unique associations between past and present experiences. GLPs provide the most joyful and rewarding moments for a therapist or a parent when we truly see one another, get one another, value one another.

We meet a child's sensory and movement needs

In our sessions, children move when they need to, enjoy their sensory experiences and take time to process sensory information. They will often show us when they need quiet, when they need space to think. Autistic children are deeply calming to be around if their sensory needs are being met and they are absorbed in an activity of their choosing that allows them to explore their enthusiasms. We will learn more about how we might help a child to meet their sensory needs and help them to up-regulate or down-regulate in Chapter 10.

A dysregulated child will not be able to communicate. We enable children to meet their sensory and movement needs, and we observe how communication then flows.

Child-led, play-based

Language acquisition occurs in natural communication contexts that are child-led and play-based. This goes for older GLPs too. We observe their sensory interests, their enthusiasms, their preferences, and we join in.

This includes use of media. If a child loves watching certain YouTube clips and rewinds and rewatches the same segment over and over, we join them in this. We might copy back the language associated with the clip, mimicking the exact intonation.

We look at what a child does when they are given free choice. This is where we start. We join them.

There will be boundaries that we put in place, particularly around safety. We will word this in a way that does not set up a power dynamic: we are subject to such rules too. For example, we say, 'we can't go upstairs', or 'that's not ours'.

Space to move

Marge Blanc has described[2] how important movement is for non-speaking or minimally speaking children, in order to facilitate deeper breathing, leading to phonation in laughter or joyful vocalisations. If a child has limited speech or limited vocalisation, we may want to start with movement, and so we will need a space in which we can run, jump, climb, bounce, swing, spin, throw balls, crash into the walls, hide under furniture, crawl on hands and knees. . . .

We can create these physical spaces in a child's living room or our therapy room. We can use a gym ball or peanut ball to roll on. We might improvise a space to crawl through, like a table with a blanket thrown over it. We might add some obstacles to walk bare-footed over: cushions, bean-bags, a swimming noodle or some skittles. We might hide objects up high or down low, so that the child has to reach and develop their core strength, which will support their phonation and sustained vocalisations.

Honouring the child's play

We start with just observing the child's play. This may not look like conventional, neurotypical play. It may involve close inspection of objects; sniffing or tasting; pressing items to the face. It may be highly physical: running, jumping, hopping, bouncing, climbing, sliding, rolling, crawling; squeezing into spaces; crashing into cushions. It might look or sound like 'stimming': spinning, rocking, flicking fingers in front of their face; peering through their finger; making loud or quiet vocalisations; humming, singing or reciting scripts.

If we are struggling to connect with a child, we probably need to start where they are at with their play, and show them that we value it. We offer them more opportunities to play in this way, perhaps offering similar experiences. If they like fluff, we offer other items with a soft texture, say feathers, pom-poms or wool. If they like throwing, we offer sensory balls or beanbags, or make a game of throwing items so that they make a noise.

Many children enjoy games of 'peekaboo' or 'I'm gonna get you', or routines which involve a predictable surprise. We might offer a new routine, but we are not demanding compliance or waiting for a particular response. If a child finds it delightful, we do it again. If they don't, we show them that we have noted their play preference. We are not trying to be a children's entertainer, but an attuned, respectful communication partner. We are building trust.

Those therapists who are trained in Intensive Interaction will find this part familiar. We are joining the person in their sensory motor world, and learning about what is interesting about the activity. We value the person's activity. We do not try to change what they are doing: where they are at right now is valued.

Different children will have different play schema preferences. Some will love taking things out of containers. Some will enjoy stacking, some will enjoy lining objects up or arranging them. We respect these, and we don't try to change them.

Gestalt processors may try to recreate whole experiences through their play. If there are sequences of actions or certain routines that they are creating, we will want to partner with a parent to identify where this has come from and what it might mean. If we are already a trusted communication partner, the child will likely give us a few clues.

Young people and adults can still play. There is a lot of worry about age-appropriate interests. Adults with autism tell us that they have felt shamed into letting go of 'childish' interests before they were ready. A therapeutic relationship is based on trust and mutual respect. We can invite the person to bring items from home into sessions, and treat them with the reverence and curiosity that they deserve.

Embracing a child's enthusiasms

In his book and associated podcast 'Uniquely Human',[3] Barry Prizant celebrates the enthusiasms of autistic and neurodivergent people. Enthusiasms are a source of great joy, and so perfect for sharing in play sessions. We are likely to foster engagement if we bring in dinosaurs or rocket ships, big cats, numbers, letters or logos, as appropriate for an individual. We can use favourite books or video clips that feature Dr Who or Star Wars. If we are working with a child or young person in their usual environment, we will have access to items associated with their enthusiasms. If we are in a school or clinic environment, we might ask a parent to bring a favourite toy or two.

Enthusiasms change. Autistic people may delve into a subject into such depth that they exhaust its interest and move on. We will need to move on when they do.

Bilingual and multilingual language acquisition

We always promote the child's home languages, and work with parents and relevant interpreters. Code-switching is a natural part of multilingual development. Just as we would never insist a child only uses one mode of communication, we would never expect them to use one language throughout an interaction. Multilingual language acquisition offers a richness of sound sources that may be particularly delightful for GLPs. This is a rich seam for current and future research. See the 'Natural Communication' and 'Communication Development Center' websites for more information about bilingual and multilingual language acquisition, including handouts that have been translated into different languages.

Recommended toys and equipment

There is no recommended list of toys or equipment. This is a highly flexible approach, which is child-led, and so the favourite activities will depend upon the child. However there are certain pieces of equipment and toys that I have found especially useful, and these are as follows:

Therapy ball or peanut ball

Sensory balls

A blanket for making dens over a table

Bags or boxes of interesting objects to discover

Musical instruments

Items to sort or arrange

Marble run

Wind-up toys, especially animals that move in different ways

Duplo, Lego or Magnet tiles

Kinetic sand, play-dough, gloop or cornflour paste

Cars or trains with roads or tracks

Wooden or plastic food with pots and pans

Animal figures or mini figures

Board books, Lift-the-Flap books

Drawing and writing equipment

Magnetic letters or numbers and a board

Everything that the child does is meaningful

This approach assumes communicative intent. The child may not be signalling this in a conventional way. They may be cautious in engaging people, because of past experiences where demands were placed that they were not ready for.

One of the most impactful aspects of this approach, particularly for older children, is that we recognise that they are communicating.

We need to get to know a child and allow them to trust us. To do this, we will not rush them into communication. We will not make demands on them to engage with us. We will likely observe them initially. If we can see that our presence unsettles them, we will keep our distance. The child may have had experience of well-meaning adults being intrusive, stepping in too early and trying to guide them into interaction that they were not ready for. This approach can be deeply healing for children and their parents if they have experienced compliance-based approaches.

We model language, but only when we have connection

Obviously we are here because we want the child to acquire language. But before language comes connection. The most primary communication function is to foster connection.

It is helpful to know what stage of Natural Language Acquisition a child is mostly living in. We can somewhat tailor our language modelling to their stage. But we are not consciously modelling language all of the time. A child would feel our hidden agenda! Whatever stage of NLA a child is in, we just talk naturally for at least 50% of the time. This is true of therapy, and for other adults supporting a child at home or in school.

We are looking to immerse the child in a communication environment that sees them, hears them, is listening deeply and is also here to keep them company and have some fun along the way.

Natural language

We try to use child-friendly language that the child's speaking peers are using. We will try to make it appealing for this child. We will try to notice if they like highly musical language with rich intonation. We might use fun voices, if the language that they are picking up from media is using fun voices. This is all an exploration: what is appealing to one child will not be the same for another.

We don't know which phrases will stick. We do not ever cue them or prompt them. There are no fixed choices, no sentence-completions. We are offering language, and the child will pick it up if they are ready. Some phrases will stick, some won't.

Taught language is forced language. It may be done very gently and in a supportive manner. But it is still forced. So we won't use prompts like 'ready . . . steady . . .' or sentence starters like 'I want . . . '. We won't offer forced alternatives. We won't withhold a toy or delay a fun action, waiting for a predefined word or phrase from a child. Forced language tends not to stick. The child may be able to produce it on demand in that situation in order to please the adult, but rarely will they use it spontaneously in other situations.

We pay attention to our own regulation

We need to be aware of co-regulation. If we are dysregulated through stress and anxiety about our own performance, we will unwittingly help to dysregulate a child.

Video can be our critical friend here. If we video our sessions we can see when we are talking too much, or doing too much, from anxiety.

Co-regulation is a domino effect. When one person in the room is dysregulated, they quickly infect everyone with this. Of course, there may be times when the child has become so relaxed that we might want to wake them up and get them moving. Video can help us identify a child's response to our energy levels, and vice versa.

Language samples are our assessment

Traditional assessment tools do not work for Gestalt Language Processors. We cannot assess receptive language though key-word assessment. We cannot used standardised assessments. These are geared towards analytic language development. It would be impossible for us to accurately assess a GLP's receptive language using formal assessments, because their understanding of the world is so personal, so nuanced and so gestalt!

Our assessment starts with information we get from the parent. They can tell us about the child's history of language exposure, the child's chosen communication modes, their current language, their sensory and movement and play preferences, how they navigate the world about them and any challenges they are having.

Our language samples are our main form of assessment, but we need to get to know a child in order to get good information from a language sample. Parents can help us out by sending us home video clips, or taking language samples at home. Language samples allow us to track a child's progression through the stages of NLA. They guide our supports for each stage of NLA, and identify any gaps in the variety of language.

If a child is non-speaking or minimally speaking, we can still take multi-modal communication samples (see the multimodal language sample in the handouts section). For each interactive turn, the message (or the possible communication intention) and the mode of communication are noted, and these then can also be scored within the NLA framework.

Is therapy needed?

Many GLPs and dual processors (those who use both gestalt and analytic strategies) will never need to see a Speech and Language Therapist. They will progress through the stages and become competent communicators. Other children will benefit from a parent-coaching model where the SLT supports a parent and teaching staff through the child's Natural Language Acquisition, perhaps helping to make suggestions for play, communication and language modelling.

Some children will benefit from direct one-to-one therapy sessions with an NLA-informed Speech and Language Therapist. If a parent feels that their child is not progressing through the stages, if the child is minimally speaking or non-speaking, or if a child's speech is highly unintelligible, they will likely seek the support of an SLT.

Therapy sessions will look very much like play. The therapist will start by observing and building trust. They will be sensitive to the preferences of the child. Once trust and connection have been established, the therapist will be alive to play experiences that will be memorable and meaningful for the child, and will judiciously model language to accompany these moments. The therapist will video the sessions and collect regular language samples (from home and within sessions), and share these with the parent and teaching staff. The therapist will make recommendations for how to support the child in their natural environment so that they are able to progress through the stages of language acquisition.

The child will want to come to therapy sessions. They know that there is a treasure trove of experiences and an adult who is there to share in these experiences.

The parent may be present, and there will ideally be cross-fertilisation of ideas between therapist and parent about what is most engaging for the child right now. If the parent does not attend because the session is school-based, then there will be a way of sharing insights and tracking language together. This might be through a shared document or sending video clips, with the parents' consent and through a secure channel.

Each child will throw up interesting clinical questions. Having an informed group of peers to consult with is essential for the SLT. There are many NLA peer support groups online, and I also recommend starting a local peer supervision group.

Having established the foundational principles of NLA, the next few chapters will focus on each stage of Natural Language Acquisition.

Notes

1 Bascom, J. (ed.) (2012) *Loud Hands: Autistic People, Speaking* The Autistic Press.
2 Blanc, M. (2006) 'Finding the words . . . when it's hard to find your voice' *Autism and Asperger's Digest*, January–February.
3 Prizant, B. & Fields-Meyer, T. (2022) *Uniquely Human: A Different Way of Seeing Autism (Revised and Expanded)* Souvenir Press.

Chapter 4

Taking and scoring a language sample

You may want to skip this chapter for now and read all about the stages of NLA before you think about scoring a language sample. This is a chapter that we will come back to again and again. Scoring a language sample takes practice, and there are many nuances. This chapter covers stage 1–4 scoring. Chapters 8 and 9 deal with stages 4–6 in detail, as we start to use a tool called Developmental Sentence Scoring (DSS).

This is our assessment

Language samples are our assessment using the NLA framework. We focus upon expressive language because this is the part of language development that we can measure. Receptive language is very difficult to assess for GLPs, particularly before they reach stage 3 of NLA, because until stage 3 they are not referential. They do have profound understanding, but it is not easy to quantify or describe.

What does a language sample show us?

Language samples allow us to:

- Show a child's communication competence. From stage 1 we can show how they are trying to connect with others.

- Track a child's progress as they acquire new gestalts in stage 1. We partner with parents to find out where they came from and what they might mean.

- Track themes or topics that are particularly important for the child. This will help us be more attuned communication partners.

- Track a child's communication intentions, so that if needed, we can model phrases to cover a wider range of communication intentions.

- Track a child's use of mitigations in stage 2. When we have tracked their stage 1 gestalts we can more easily identify stage 2 mitigations.

- Identify when a child is entering the referential stage 3. We especially need to check that these are true stage 3 isolations of nouns, attributes and locations.

DOI: 10.4324/9781032717029-4

- Track the variety in their stage 3 language: that a range of semantic relationships are being explored in word + word combinations.

- Identify when a child is entering stage 4 and is starting to use self-generated grammar.

- Identify any 'mini-chunks' that may need further breaking down, e.g. contractions like 'we're' and 'isn't' or word combinations like 'that one' or 'no more'.

- Identify the grammatical language structures that we need to model in stages 5 and 6.

- Analyse the percentage of utterances in each stage of NLA, in order to provide appropriate language modelling.

- Write detailed reports which show progress over a course of therapy or school year.

- Write appropriate goals for therapy and informative reports for parents and schools.

Prior to taking a first language sample

Some useful questions to ask parents are:

- What languages has your child been exposed to?

- Do they show a preference for any particular language?

- What are their favourite things to do?

- What sensory experiences or movements do they enjoy?

- What do they like to watch or listen to?

- Do they have any favourite toys?

- Do they have any favourite books or stories?

- Have you noticed any echoed language (from other people, from songs, from video clips, from stories)?

- What are their current modes of communication? e.g. hand-leading, speech, sign, pointing, leading, vocalisations, AAC, sharing media clips, reading or spelling.

- How do they like to play?

- Do they reenact scenes from tv or movies in their play?

- Do they enjoy writing or drawing? (even if it is not recognisable as writing yet)

- What Speech and Language Therapy have they had before?

- Have they used PECS or symbolised supports?

- What does your child need in order to thrive?

- What do you love most about your child?

This information will give us some useful background information so that we know roughly what to expect in our first language sample.

As part of my research for writing this book, I heard from therapists who carry out consultative work in preschools and schools, who have managed to carry out child-led sessions and take a language sample without this background information. They have then checked in with a parent and the parent has been able to help them refine their language sample scoring.

How do we take a language sample?

We will not get our best language sample from the first session. This is likely to come once we have established a relationship with a child.

We will provide a child-led play-based session. Ideally the space will allow room to move around, and there will be play equipment and toys that we know the child likes.

We want to get a natural language sample. We will say and do what is needed to keep the conversation going. We don't prompt the child or ask questions that require an answer. If the child speaks, we will respond positively, acknowledging their communication intention in a way we know they like. For some children this may be a nod or a vocalisation to encourage them. It might sometimes mean repeating back what they say. We might say something to keep the conversation going, taking their train of thought and adding to it.

If the child's speech is unintelligible, we will acknowledge it with a warm face and an encouraging vocalisation. We might try to interpret their communication intention and respond accordingly.

If the child is saying a lot, we can say more to respond to their language. We try to match the complexity of their language, and only if they are obviously in stage 5 or beyond will we use longer sentences.

We don't ask questions when we are taking a language sample. Many autistic children are used to being asked formulaic questions, and many may have acquired the 'correct' response. We want to show the child that we will not make language demands on them. We are here to partner them in this process; to enjoy being with them and to learn from them.

We are aiming to capture 50 spontaneous utterances, or a language sample of at least 12 minutes. Fifty utterances give us a large enough sample to score the different stages, and then to be confident that this is reflective of their everyday language.

Video is the best way to take a language sample, as it also captures non-speech communication. We can then transcribe the language sample, using a template included in the handouts section.

It is recommended that we take a language sample at least every three to six weeks. We are not only looking at the relative prevalence of language from each stage, but also the variety in language, and in communication intentions. In later stages, we will be looking at grammatical constructions and noting any mini-chunks that need to be further broken down.

Our language samples can incorporate language that a parent has heard at home or that a teaching assistant has heard in school. In fact this gives us valuable information about the breadth of language being used in different situations.

As much as is practical, we want a verbatim transcription of what the child said, with all linguistic errors or omissions, quirks of word order or semantic and pragmatic use. It's all useful information. We also transcribe the communication partner's contributions, so that we can see if there is any immediate echolalia. This would be scored as 'o' in the language sample.

What does each stage of language sound like?

Stage 1

- Stage 1 gestalts are the soundtracks to an experience. They are unanalysed wholes: the original 'unit of meaning' as described by Ann Peters.

- They might be unintelligible strings of babble or intonational curves with vowels and semivowels.

- Stage 1 gestalts may also be heard phrases, songs, lines from books or YouTube clips, or longer scripts. As a child gets older and their speech develops, their stage 1 gestalts will get clearer.

- Stage 1 gestalts may be accompanied by actions. They may be stories or scripts which are physically acted out.

- Older children may have extremely long gestalts because they have had more time to memorise long scripts.

- Stage 1 gestalts may also be single words. If the child has heard adults label a lot of items, colours and numbers, there may be a lot of single word gestalts. Listen out for the word being said with the same intonational contour each time, or the same voice quality. If we only hear a single word in isolation and never hear it as part of a longer construction, it may have become stuck as a single word gestalt.

Stage 2

- Once we are familiar with a child's stage 1 gestalts, it will be easier to identify stage 2 language. We will recognise a chunk that has been trimmed down from a stage 1 gestalt. We will recognise a 'frame-and-slot' construction that has evolved from the original gestalt.

- Early stage 2 language is likely to have retained the original intonational contour in the trimmed-down chunk. This is a clue that it is a stage 2 mitigation, rather than a self-generated stage 4 phrase or sentence.

- Single words may also be stage 2 mitigations: trimmed down from a longer gestalt. This is really hard to spot when we are first getting to know a child. If we don't know their language well, it is safer to score single words as stage 1 until we have evidence that they are stage 2 or 3.

- Sometimes a gestalt may be mitigated by the intonational curve changing. For example, the phrase 'it's mine!' has always been produced with falling intonation but is now produced with a questioning intonation pattern: 'it's mine?' This would be classed as a stage 2 mitigation, because the gestalt has changed from the original.

- Stage 2 mitigations may get trimmed down and trimmed down until a single word is isolated. Until we hear that isolated word in a new word + word combination, we will code it as a stage 2 mitigation.

Stage 3

- Stage 3 is entered when stage 2 mitigations have been trimmed down to isolated words and that word is then also seen in a word + word combination.

- Stage 3 consists of isolated nouns, attributes or locations, and word + word combinations of these elements. They are referential, and literal. The entry into stage 3 is likely to be accompanied by pointing, showing or matching.

- There may be a hesitancy or a flatness of tone in stage 3 language, marking a change from the rich intonation of stage 1 and stage 2 language.

- Word order is fluid in stage 3. This is the referential stage, not the grammar stage. We might hear (and model) 'banana . . . yellow' and 'yellow . . . banana'. Stage 4 is the start of grammar, and a more fixed word order.

Stage 4

- We may see linguistic dysfluency (also known as 'mazing') in stage 4 language. For the first time, the child is actively searching for the next word to put into the phrase or sentence. There is a huge burden on their language processing, and therefore we will see some dysfluency: hesitancy, repetitions and maybe 'fillers'.

- Stage 4 language is experimental grammar. We will see word order beginning to be more important, but initially there will be errors in word order and there will be limited morphology.

- Stage 4 is a huge stage. Early stage 4 phrases and sentences are short and simple, but by the end of stage 4 there are early verb tenses, plurals, negatives and questions. We will recognise a stage 4 utterance by knowing the child's stage 1 and 2 language well.

- Unless they are in stage 1, a GLP child will have a mixture of stages at any one time. They are naturally drawn to the whole, so they will go on acquiring gestalts and then breaking them down. This process will become more efficient as they move through the stages.

Multiple languages

If a child uses multiple languages, we will partner with the family to help us transcribe language samples. Code-switching is a natural part of multilingual development. Just as we would never insist a child only uses one mode of communication, we would never expect them to use one language throughout an interaction. We will need to enlist the help of the family and/or an interpreter in charting a phrase's journey from stage 1 to stage 2 and beyond. This is a rich seam of current and future research, and practitioners are encouraged to share their experiences and language samples with the various NLA study groups (see the 'Communication Development Center' and 'Natural Communication' websites for more information).

Multi-modal communication

Some children will use mainly speech (mouth-words), but others may use modalities such as Makaton signs, communication boards or books or communication apps on an iPad. If they are using language across different modalities, try to specify this in your language sample. An utterance may use multiple modes, and so capture this in your language sample too. A template is provided for a 'Multi-modal (AAC) language sample' in the handouts section.

What if the child only uses echolalia?

If we can understand the language, then transcribe this. If it is largely unintelligible, then we can note this. The convention is to use xxx for unintelligible words or utterances. If there are recognisable words within the stream of echolalia, we try to capture these: they will be useful for the detective work to find out where the gestalt came from and what it means. We can even mark the syllables in a gestalt, and possibly the intonation pattern. Echoed phrases stay true to the origin of the gestalt: the same intonation pattern is used every time. The child will likely use the same pronunciation or dialect of the original gestalt. The musicality and voice quality are important: they may give us a clue where the gestalt came from. If the gestalt is a song, try to capture it, even if it is the first line.

Echolalic children sometimes speak very quietly, because they have become habituated to their language not being acknowledged or understood. They may use a very high-pitched voice, or a very low-pitched voice. We are more likely to be able to hear them if we are very quiet ourselves. We need to show them that we are listening.

If a child is using a long script, we may find that it gets louder or slower or more insistent at the important part: this is because the child has recognised that this is the phrase they need. They aren't yet able to trim down that gestalt (that is for stage 2), but they have recognised the part that they want us to listen to.

Immediate echolalia versus delayed echolalia

Immediate echolalia is where a child repeats what we have just modelled. Immediate echolalia will be scored as 'o' in our language samples. This is not because it is unimportant. It is an important part of any child's language acquisition. They are building the motor pathways for phonation, constructing syllables and extracting chunks from the sound-stream. They are taking turns and learning about the to-and-fro of conversation. As children move through NLA stages, we may find that they can copy back a new chunk of language and then immediately mitigate it, and even isolate the important word and use it in a self-generated construction. Immediate echolalia continues to be useful.

Delayed echolalia is a stage 1 gestalt. This is the child's Natural Language Acquisition: the language that they have saved for later, to be used in new contexts.

This is the language that will be trimmed down, split into chunks and recombined in stage 2.

'Taught' language

It may be that a child has been taught single words like 'more' and 'biscuit' and phrases such as 'I want biscuit'. They may have lots of taught language: the adult says a prompt, and the child knows what is expected of them.

This is taught language, and is not their Natural Language Acquisition. It has been elicited.

A well-intentioned adult may have offered single word modelling. They may have offered a choice and waited for the child to give a single word response. They may have trained the child to say a phrase, either with speech or pictures or symbols.

Taught language often has a particular auditory quality. It sounds empty of emotion or meaning. It sounds dull. It differs dramatically from gestalt language. Gestalt sounds more engaged and emotionally charged. It is a GLP's 'love language' and is therefore more exciting!

We score taught language as 'o'. If this word or phrase has been specifically taught, or targeted, then this is not natural language. The child would not have naturally picked up this language had it not been prompted until the child said what was expected.

Older children, particularly those who have received PECS or ABA input, are likely to have some taught language. Look out for the classic 'I want' and 'I see' phrases.

What if the child does not speak?

If a normally speaking child becomes non-speaking when we attempt to take a language sample, we could ask the parent to send us audio or video recordings of them, to get a more representative sample. If a child is dysregulated because this is a totally new setting with a new person, they may be quieter than normal.

It is estimated that 25–30% of autistic children are minimally or non-speaking,[1] and so it is entirely possible that we will have a child who does not speak at all in the whole session.

If a child is completely silent, this is still important information for our assessment. We will watch the video recording carefully and note other modes of communication. See the 'Multi-modal (AAC) language sample' template in the handouts section. There is likely to be non-verbal communication: changes in breathing, body proximity (or distancing), leaning forward or backing away, facial expressions or eye-gaze, hand-leading and so on. All of this information is valid: it shows that the child is communicating.

If a child is minimally or non-speaking, we will need to consider movement, and the possible part that AAC might need to play in the child's language acquisition. See Chapter 11 for more information about speech and Chapter 12 for more information on AAC for GLPs.

What if we don't get 50 utterances?

The gold standard for a language sample is 50 spontaneous, unprompted utterances, with the adult just doing enough to keep the interaction going (by saying 'uh huh', repeating the child's phrases and maybe sometimes adding to them).

If we don't get 50 utterances, we may ask the parent to record the child's language at other times. Our 50 utterances may come from three or four separate recordings, but as long as they are recorded in a limited time period, of about a week, we can be confident that we have a snapshot of that child's current language.

If the child doesn't produce much language, then we use what we've got. Bear in mind that this is not the ideal scenario and so our conclusions are speculative and less certain than they would be with a 50 utterance sample. A language sample of 20 utterances is probably the absolute minimum that will allow us to calculate the percentages in each stage, and we will check our instincts and the parents' instincts for whether this feels representative.

Scoring a language sample

Scoring a language sample using the NLA framework takes practice. At first this seems like an overwhelming task, but, like scoring a standardised test, it becomes easier with practice.

The first language sample for a new child is the hardest to score, but familiarity with the child makes each subsequent language sample easier to score. Parents are our partners, and their input is vital when deciding whether a phrase is a gestalt. Once we become more familiar with the child's gestalts, our scoring starts to flow. We can more easily recognise a stage 2 mitigation from a recognised gestalt.

The following are the basics of scoring a language sample. We will need to refer to this many times before scoring becomes automatic and intuitive. It is helpful to discuss our scoring with another SLT who has familiarity with NLA. We can seek peer supervision to check our scoring.

It is important to note that the same utterance could be scored at different stages. It depends upon our knowledge of the child's language.

1. Immediate echolalia is scored 'o'. So if the adult says, 'we can swing high!' and the child repeats 'we can swing high' or 'swing high!' we score this as o.

2. If the child later uses this phrase, we score it as stage 1. It has been retained and reused meaningfully as a stage 1 gestalt.

3. Whole phrases that are always said in the same way with the same intonation pattern are stage 1. This includes lines from songs and books, movie scripts, overheard phrases and modelled stage 1 phrases.

4. Single words can also be stage 1. The single word has been acquired as a gestalt. We never hear the child combining this word with other words. It has been processed by the child as a whole (a gestalt).

5. If a gestalt starts to be trimmed down, it is a stage 2 mitigation. For example, if the original gestalt was the line of a song 'what do you see? What do you see? I see a stegosaurus!' but then we hear 'I see a stegosaurus' on its own, this is a stage 2 mitigation.

6. If there is a 'frame-and-slot' construction, it is a stage 2 mitigation. For example, the original gestalt is 'here come the babies!' but now we hear 'here come the . . . mummy!' it is a stage 2 mitigation.

7. If two gestalts are 'mix-and-matched' it is a stage 2 mitigation. For example, if we hear 'here come the . . . stegosaurus' or 'I see a . . . cheeky monkey'.

8. If a gestalt has been trimmed and trimmed until the child uses a single word from an original gestalt, the single word is scored as stage 2 until we hear it in an original word + word stage 3 combination.

9. Single words are only scored as stage 3 if they have been isolated from a stage 1 or stage 2 utterance. We are cautious with our stage 3 scoring until we can be sure this is a referential word. Stage 3 language is often accompanied by pointing, showing or matching.

10. Word + word combinations are only scored as stage 3 if we have heard each word in isolation too. For the phrase 'duck . . . orange' to be scored as

stage 3, we would have to have heard 'duck' in isolation and we would have to have heard 'orange' in isolation.

11. Stage 3 is the 'slowing down and taking a pause' stage. This is the first time that the GLP is using referential language. It is the first time that they have realised that the word represents a fixed meaning. That is a huge shift. Their language might switch from fluent and free-flowing and richly intonational stage 1 gestalts and stage 2 mitigations, to stilted single words and word + word combinations. It can sound slow and strange, and surprising, not least to the child themselves. There is often a pause between the words in word + word combinations, at least early in stage 3.

12. Stage 3 consists of nouns, attributes and locations. These are the more concrete, referential units of language. The child is almost checking with you that this thing that they are pointing to is 'apple' or 'little'.

13. The word order is free in stage 3. We might hear 'dog . . . big' or 'big . . . dog', 'dog . . . bird' or 'bird . . . dog'.

14. Stage 4 encompasses other word types and other word combinations. It includes the modifiers 'more', 'no', 'this', 'that'. It includes verbs like 'is', 'got', 'jump' and 'sleep'. Examples of stage 4 are 'more car', 'this big', 'me got car' and 'it jump'.

15. Stage 4 includes pre-sentences (phrases) and early experimental sentences.

16. Stage 4 initially resembles telegraphic speech, with few grammatical morphemes, and overgeneralisation of grammatical rules.

17. Contractions like 'we're' and 'let's' may still appear as 'mini-chunks' in stage 4. We note their presence, and model the separate words.

18. There may also be mini-chunks of word combinations that always appear together. For example, '(find it) pizza' or '(get it) that one'. If we see mini-chunks, we put brackets around them. We know we need to model these words separately to help to isolate them.

19. We will get to stages 5 and 6 in Chapter 9. For now, we will focus on stages 1–4.

20. If an utterance is unintelligible, we will not score this. It will be included in our language sample, but we don't score it.

21. We allocate each scoreable utterance a number, so that we can easily refer to each utterance if we are discussing the scoring with a parent or a colleague. If we have a full language sample, we will have at least 50 numbered utterances.

Calculating the percentage of utterances at each NLA stage

Once we have scored each utterance, we can calculate the percentage of utterances in each NLA stage.

- First calculate the total number of utterances that we have scored. Let's say this is 50.

- Then count up the number of utterances in each stage. For example:

    Stage 1: 23

    Stage 2: 18

    Stage 3: 9

    Stage 4: 0

- To calculate the percentage of utterances in stage 1, divide the number of utterances in stage 1 by the total number of utterances, and then multiply by 100. Do the same for stages 2, 3 and 4.

    Stage 1: 46%

    Stage 2: 36%

    Stage 3: 18%

    Stage 4: 0%

1. If 80% or more of the utterances in an appropriate sample are at one stage, the child is very much 'living in this stage'.

2. If 50% or more of the utterances in an appropriate sample are at one stage, the child is likely operating at that stage most of the time.

3. If no single stage is represented more than 50% of the time, then processes at more than one stage are being used.

4. In that scenario, the highest stage that is represented in the language sample suggests that the child is developing towards that stage.

How this informs our language modelling

Our aim is to use natural language at least 50% of the time. We will just be trying to be with the child, and keep the conversation going.

Knowing which stage a child is predominantly 'living in' will guide us when we are intentionally modelling language for a child. We are thinking about what language will be useful for the child next.

Table 4.1 describes what supports a child might benefit from, depending on the scored language sample.

Table 4.1 Language supports at different stages of NLA

If the language sample shows:	Then we can:
Stage 1	
If the child is using stage 1 language more than 50% of the time, and has not yet used any mitigations . . .	Model appealing phrases in the child's chosen modality that can be easily mitigated.
If the child is using stage 1 language for 25–50% of the time, plus language from later stages . . .	Look at the variety in their stage 2 mitigations. What other mitigations might be useful? Do they need some more stage 1 language that can then be mitigated?
If the child is using stage 1 language less than 25% of the time, plus language from later stages . . .	Stage 1 language is likely the 'background' for later stage language. The child will continue to acquire new gestalts naturally.
Stage 2	
If the child is using stage 2 language more than 50% of the time . . .	Provide lots of social opportunities for the child to use their stage 2 language. This will support more flexible use of mitigations, and will help prepare for stage 3.
If the child is using stage 2 language for 25–50% of the time . . .	Look at the variety in their stage 2 mitigations. Continue to model new stage 1 and 2 language. Use their mitigations and model new possibilities.
If the child is using stage 2 language less than 25% of the time . . .	Look at the variety in the child's stage 1 gestalts and mitigations. Provide more variety in stage 1 if needed, and more examples of mitigation.

(Continued)

If the language sample shows:	Then we can:
Stage 3	
If the child is starting to use some stage 3 language . . .	Provide opportunities to practice this in referencing games, e.g. pointing to items, comparing or matching them, describing them, hiding and finding them.
If the child is using stage 3 language for more than 50% of the time . . .	Look at the variety of nouns, attributes and locations, and the variety of semantic relationships being expressed. Provide opportunities to explore the full range (see Chapter 7 for details)
If the child is using stage 3 language for 25–50% of the time . . .	As above. The child may also need more stage 2 language to break down to create this variety in stage 3.
If the child is using stage 3 language for less than 25% of the time . . .	Look at the other stages represented in the language sample. If the child is using stage 2 flexibly and well plus a small amount of stage 3, this may be sufficient for stage 4 development.
Stage 4	
If the child is using stage 4 (or higher) for more than 50% of the time . . .	Examine the language sample for types of grammatical construction. Incorrect constructions give as much information as correct constructions. If the child has not gone through a stage of grammatical errors, it may be that they are using scripted stage 2 sentences. If these do seem to be self-generated, model any new constructions that may be needed. The child's natural play will likely provide inspiration for this.

(Continued)

If the language sample shows:	Then we can:
If the child is using stage 4–6 for 25–50% of the time . . .	Look at DST combinations for variety (see Chapters 7 and 8), and model more variety if needed. Also look at the variety of vocabulary represented. We may need to create opportunities to talk in a wide range of settings and with different play opportunities to inspire wide variety in vocabulary and grammar.
If the child is using stage 4–6 less than 25% of the time . . .	Examine the language sample for other stages. If there is not sufficient variety in stage 1, 2 or 3, then this will limit stage 4 development. Create memorable experiences to promote further language growth in earlier stages.

Language sample scoring: examples

I will now take you through the scoring of some language samples, enlisting the help of 4-year-old GLP, Jack. For simplicity, I have only included Jack's utterances in the language samples. In a full language sample, I would include the communication partner's utterances. I have also restricted each sample to around ten utterances: any more would have resulted in a very long chapter!

Table 4.2 Language sample 1

Utterance	NLA Stage	Explanation
mummy do it!	1	This is a phrase that Jack uses when he needs help. It is always said with the same intonation pattern.
What's this?	1	This is a phrase that Jack uses when he discovers something new.

(Continued)

Utterance	NLA Stage	Explanation
Five little monkeys jumping on the bed. One fell off and bumped his head!	1	This is a song that Jack sings when he is bouncing or making a toy bounce.
I did it!	0	I modelled this first, and Jack copied it back. For now it is scored as 0. If I hear it spontaneously later, it will be scored as 1.
It's a dinosaur!	0	As above
cat	1	I have not heard this word in combination with another noun, attribute or location, and so for now I will score this as a 1. GLPs can often pick up a lot of single words, but they are still gestalts. The child might be using the word to depict a range of meanings, e.g. 'remember when we saw that cat jump off the roof?' or 'I love fluffy animals'.
red	1	As above. Until I hear this attribute in combination with other single nouns, attributes or locations, I will score it as a stage 1 gestalt.
Mummy do it!	1	Another clue that a phrase is a stage 1 gestalt is that it recurs often. It is said with the same intonation pattern each time.
Mummy do it!	1	Stage 1 language is often quite repetitive. If we get multiples of the same gestalt, we score each one separately.
It's a dinosaur!	1	Jack has retained this phrase and used it spontaneously (rather than immediate echolalia), and so this is now scored as 1.

Table 4.3 Language sample 1 analysis

	Number of utterances	**Percentage of utterances**
Total number of utterances	10	
0	2	20
Stage 1	8	80
Stage 2	0	0
Stage 3	0	0
Stage 4	0	0

In this language sample (Table 4.3), there is no language above stage 1, and so we are confident that Jack is currently living in stage 1. We will take more language samples in the coming weeks, to track the variety of stage 1 language. For now we assume he needs more stage 1 language, because he is not naturally mitigating yet.

Table 4.4 Language sample 2

Utterance	**NLA stage**	**Explanation**
Mummy do it!	1	I have got to know this as a stage 1 gestalt.
Jack do it	0	Jack's mum modelled this and Jack copied it, so for now I am scoring it as 0.
Five little monkeys jumping on the bed. One fell off and bumped his head!	1	Songs are a natural way for Jack to acquire new language.

(Continued)

Utterance	NLA stage	Explanation
It's a dinosaur!	1	This is the gestalt acquired in the previous session. It is said with the same intonation pattern every time.
It's a helicopter!	2	This is the first time I have heard a mitigation. Jack is using the frame of 'it's a . . .' with a new noun slotted in.
We've got chocolate ice cream!	0	This was repeated after my modelling, so for now it is 0.
It's a mummy!	2	This is another stage 2 mitigation.
helicopter	2	This may be a stage 3 word, but I cannot be sure yet. I need to hear it both in isolation and in combination with another noun, or with an attribute or location. I am suspecting Jack is heading in this direction, because this word has been isolated from the stage 2 mitigation 'it's a helicopter!'
triangle	1	As above
green	1	As above

Table 4.5 Language sample 2 analysis

	Number of utterances	**Percentage of utterances**
Total number of utterances	10	
0	2	20
Stage 1	5	50
Stage 2	3	30
Stage 3	0	0
Stage 4	0	0

In this language sample (Tables 4.4 and 4.5), Jack has started mitigating. He is 50% at stage 1 and 30% at stage 2. Our priority is to keep the conversation flowing, to model more stage 1 language to provide sufficient variety, and to take his mitigations and add more variations to these, where this feels natural.

Table 4.6 Language sample 3

Utterance	**NLA stage**	**Explanation**
It's a dinosaur!	1	The original stage 1 gestalt, said with rich intonation.
It's a aeroplane!	2	Stage 2 mitigation. Note that Jack does not say 'it's an aeroplane', which is what an adult would say. This is an important clue that this is his own self-generated stage 2.
green dinosaur	3	By now I have heard both 'green' and 'dinosaur' in isolation. Jack is entering stage 3.

(Continued)

Utterance	NLA stage	Explanation
I did it!	1	I am still hearing a lot of stage 1 gestalts, and I am still modelling new stage 1 gestalts because I want to be sure that Jack has enough mitigable gestalts to set him up well for stages 2 and 3.
What's that noise?	1	Always said with the same intonation pattern.
cat	1	I have not heard this word in combination with another noun, adjective or location, and so for now I will score this as a 1.
red dinosaur	3	I have heard both 'red' and 'dinosaur' in isolation, and now in combination.
Ready steady	2	This is a stage 2 mitigation where the original 'ready steady go!' is being broken down.
Five little monkeys jumping on the bed	2	This is also a stage 2 mitigation where the whole song is now being segmented. Jack's mum is also modelling variations like 'Five little bunnies jumping on the bed'.

Table 4.7 Language sample 3 analysis

	Number of utterances	Percentage of utterances
Total number of utterances	9	
Stage 1	4	44
Stage 2	3	33
Stage 3	2	22
Stage 4	0	0

In this language sample (Tables 4.6 and 4.7), Jack is showing a mix of stages, as is typical for GLPs. We still see a lot of stage 1 language, because this is Jack's natural way of acquiring language. This is useful: it gives him more material to mitigate in stage 2 and then isolate in stage 3. Until Jack is over 50% in stage 2 we will continue to model stage 2 language. This will provide variety for stage 3 and later stage 4 language.

Table 4.8 Language sample 4

Utterance	NLA stage	Explanation
got cake here	4	This is self-generated language.
It hungry	4	As above
Where are you, aeroplane?	2	This is a mitigation. I have heard the 'where are you?' frame with a few different nouns slotted in.
That's so scary!	2	This is a stage 2 mitigation from 'that's so loud!'
Aeroplane up	3	I haven't heard 'up' in isolation, but I am now confident that Jack is in stage 3.
I see triceratops	2	This has been trimmed down from a song line.
Ok, I help you!	1	A new useful stage 1 gestalt.
Help!	2	This has been freed from the original gestalt. Until I hear it in combination it will stay as stage 2. Verbs are not scored as stage 3: stage 3 is nouns, attributes and locations.
Ready steady roll	2	These stage 2 mitigations continue to be useful for later word isolation.
Ready steady catch	2	As above.

Table 4.9 Language sample 4 analysis

	Number of utterances	**Percentage of utterances**
Total number of utterances	10	
Stage 1	1	10
Stage 2	6	60
Stage 3	1	10
Stage 4	2	20

We will need to look at the variety of language in Jack's stage 2 mitigations. If there is limited variety, then we may continue to model stage 2 mitigations, or even model new stage 1 gestalts. Looking at percentages alone, Jack's language sample is suggesting that Jack may be ready for stage 3 modelling because stage 2 is secure at over 50% of the sample and he is naturally using some stage 3 language. This is accompanied by pointing or showing. We might start to experiment with some playful referencing games with him.

A note of reassurance

Scoring is much easier when we have a real child that we are getting to know. We become familiar with their stage 1 gestalts, and so we can recognise stage 2 mitigations. We exercise caution with stage 3 until we are sure that the isolated words have been heard both in isolation and in a word + word combination. Stage 3 language is nouns, attributes and locations. The other clue is that children will generally slow down in this stage. We are used to them using fluent phrases which have rich intonation. In stage 3, that intonation pattern is lost. We can hear that each word is separate. There may be a pause between the words. This is a good sign that stage 3 has begun. Another indication is that the child starts pointing: they are using referential language.

Stage 4 begins by sounding 'telegraphic', with limited morphology. As it develops, it starts to include verb tenses, plurals, negatives and even questions. We will likely see much more flexibility now, with isolated words appearing in multiple different constructions within the same language sample.

If you are feeling overwhelmed at this point, please know that this is normal and expected. Like with any new therapy approach, we begin with *one child*. We get to know their language. We learn so much from each new child we support.

How often do we take a language sample?

Whilst the gold standard is a full language sample with both partners' utterances, this is not realistic for every therapy session. We might choose to take a full language sample every few weeks, or even every three months, depending on our perceptions of the rate of change.

As therapists we need to use our own judgement. If we are seeing a child for regular therapy, we might aim to take a shorter language sample each session, perhaps transcribing either 12 minutes of utterances, or 20 utterances. Some children talk a lot, and some children may only say a handful of utterances in a whole session. Ideally, parents will also contribute, providing a sample of language that they have heard that week. In reality, we will find our own solutions, and it will vary for the different children we support.

A caveat: a stage is an artificial construct

Just as separating human beings into 'Gestalt Language Processors' and 'Analytic Language Processors' is a simplification, imposing distinct stages into a highly complex neurodevelopmental process such as language acquisition is inevitably reductive. Each child's language acquisition is unique. In clinical practice, there do seem to be observable stages, and certain language supports do seem particularly helpful at certain stages in the process. But always bear in mind that a child moves between stages even in one interaction. Our language support should not rigidly stick to a particular stage for a whole therapy session, but be responsive to the language that the child is using with us. We may have a particular stage that we are focusing on, be it modelling more potential gestalts, modelling more mitigations, playing with isolated words and word + word combinations, or listening for experimental grammar. But we can use our clinical judgement to sprinkle in supports from other stages as the need arises.

We are always aiming to talk naturally for 50% of the time. We can't go far wrong with this.

Note

1 Brignell, A., Chenausky, K. V., Song, H., Zhu, J., Suo, C. & Morgan, A. T. (2018, November 5) 'Communication interventions for autism spectrum disorder in minimally verbal children' *Cochrane Database of Systematic Review* 11.

Chapter 5

Stage 1

Language gestalts

The most important step that we can take for a GLP is to take their language seriously; to view it as important, and worth listening to. And in so doing, we think about the potential meaning that the child is trying to convey. Stage 1 language gestalts are richly nuanced and meaningful. Sometimes opaque yes, but often profound. There is deep feeling, and with this, a deep need for connection. It is our job to partner with this child, in order for us to receive their meaning, and share the moment.

The six stages of Natural Language Acquisition

It's helpful to keep seeing stage 1 in the context of future stages, so here's a reminder (Table 5.1):

Table 5.1 The six stages of Natural Language Acquisition

		Examples
Stage 1	Language gestalts (wholes, scripts, songs, language soundtracks from experiences)	Zoom zoom zoom, we're going to the moon! It's a dinosaur!
Stage 2	Mitigations: a) Shortening long gestalts b) Dividing them into chunks c) Recombining different chunks	We're going to the moon! We're going! We're going to the shops! It's an octopus!
Stage 3	Isolated single words Word + word combinations of referential single words	dinosaur; rocket dinosaur . . . big; rocket . . . up

(Continued)

DOI: 10.4324/9781032717029-5

		Examples
Stage 4	Original phrases and beginning sentences	We got dinosaur Put rocket up there
Stage 5	Original sentences with more complex grammar	I can get the dinosaurs I don't want to put my shoes on
Stage 6	Original sentences culminating in a complete grammar system	Who could have taken the dinosaurs? I've been looking for my shoes

What does stage 1 sound like?

Stage 1 language gestalts can take different forms, but essentially a language gestalt is the soundtrack that has accompanied a memorable experience. For a child with unclear speech it might sound like an intonational sound-stream, possibly with recognisable vowel and consonant elements. It may be a word, and the word is produced with the same intonation each time. It may be a recognisable phrase, sentence, or an entire song or script from a media source. It is said in the same way every time. That is, with the same ups-and-downs of intonation, the same volume or rate, and possibly in the same accent or voice quality. It may have an accompanying facial expression, gesture or action attached. GLPs are about the whole experience, so anything that was memorable and meaningful for the child may be included.

These are some examples of stage 1 gestalts:

- 'What's this?' (said in exactly the same way each time, with rising intonation, a gasping breathy voice, and a wide-eyed look of surprise)

- 'Ok, George, open your eyes!' (a script from Peppa Pig)

- '5–4–3–2–1 . . . blast off!'

- 'Ready, steady, go!' (a common gestalt that many of us learnt!)

- 'Peepo!' (possibly accompanied by actions)

- 'Achoo!' (with the head movement included)

- 'Triangle!' (Many GLPs like to learn shapes, colours, numbers and letters, and so may have a collection of these words. They are considered stage 1 if they have not developed beyond single words and have not been trimmed down from longer gestalts. GLPs can acquire single words, but they will not spontaneously start to combine single words into a phrase. We sometimes refer to these stage 1 single words as 'stuck gestalts'.)

- 'Please welcome your host, DUGGEE! Woof woof woof woof woof. So without further ado, let's meet today's team!' (This is a script from 'Hey Duggee'. When the child started saying this stage 1 gestalt, it sounded more like this: 'pi we-uh or oh, DUGGEE! Woo woo woo woo. Oh wi-ow ur-ur adoo, eh mee ooh-ay ee!')

- 'Zoom, zoom, zoom, we're going to the moon!' (from a song, used every time a toy flies through the air).

- 'How are you? I'm well thank you'. We all have language gestalts like this: chunks of language that we use wholesale. It probably reduces processing time for us, and so is an efficient way to communicate for some communication intentions.

- A stage 1 language gestalt may be very quiet and hard to recognise as 'speech'. However when we ourselves get quiet, we can sometimes realise that an apparently non-speaking child is saying things.

- Some GLPs may have whole tv episodes or movies as language gestalts. They may recite these openly, or in their heads. We may notice that they get louder at the part of the gestalt that is most meaningful for them. They may slow down at that point and really stress the important part.

- A dyspraxic child (remembering that 25–30% of autistic children are believed to have no or very limited speech) may not be able to initiate voice at the moment, or they may hum or sing songs, scripts, phrases or words. There may be clues that they are a gestalt processor though (see the following).

- A language gestalt may be in a non-speech modality. It may be expressed through Makaton signs (one sign or a sequence of signs: the clue is that it is always expressed in the same way or same order). It may be expressed through symbols or text, pointing, drawing. . . .

- A language gestalt may be multi-modal. A sequence of elements may consist of elements from different modalities, e.g. a gesture then a mime, then a Makaton sign, then finger-spelling. If this message is always sequenced in the same way, then it is a language gestalt.

Initial assessment: parents are our partners

Parents may come to us knowing that their child is a GLP. Others may not have heard about Gestalt Language Processing. If they have not come across GLP and once we start to describe the features of GLP and they start giving examples of gestalt processing in everyday life, we are likely working with a GLP child. Questions that I find useful to ask are:

- What does your child love to do most? What brings them joy?
- What activities do they most enjoy?
- Do they enjoy particular ways of moving?
- What does their play look like?
- What patterns do you notice in their play?
- What toys or objects are they most drawn to?
- What are their favourite books, songs, media clips?
- How do they show you that they love these?
- What does your child love to learn about?
- What enables your child to thrive?
- What do you love most about your child?
- Who engages your child the most, and how do they do that?

The parent and child may have already accessed speech and language support which used ALP strategies and there was limited progress. The parent may have instinctively known that the approach was not resonating with their child. This is evidence that a child is a GLP. Ask the parent about the strategies they have used and what the child's response was.

Establishing trust and connection

The most foundational communication intention is to connect, and to share a moment together. Our priority when starting to work with a GLP is to allow connection. A GLP may be used to others 'not getting them'. It is our job to try to 'get them'. A younger child may start to trust us and enjoy being with us very quickly. An older child, especially a child who has experienced compliance-based therapies where they were required to play in a certain way or produce a certain response, will take time to trust that we are not going to direct them in that way.

We will need to demonstrate that their natural play is valued. They can line up toys, keep toys to themselves, choose not to engage with toys but to bounce around the room, or stay very quiet and keep to their own space.

We will not try to be a children's entertainer. We will have a selection of play equipment that we know from the parent the child might enjoy, but if they are not inclined to play with any of this today, we are not going to try to persuade them.

The child is free to meet their sensory and movement needs: we might offer equipment that lends itself to bouncing, balancing, throwing, catching, pushing, pulling (see Chapters 10 and 11 for more on this). Provided it is not dangerous, we go with whatever the child chooses to do in the session. We are here to validate their natural choices. We are listening to and watching out for their natural communication, and this can take whatever form they choose.

We are keeping communication alive

We are here to keep connection going. We will only do what is needed to continue a child's idea or action. We will join in if they are happy for us to join in. We might occasionally offer an idea, but we will carefully observe their reaction to this. If we see that they did not like this, we note it, and we make it clear to them that we recognised our contribution was not welcome.

Therapists who are new to this approach may worry that they are not doing enough. We may feel that it feels too easy. We are in the moment, following a child's lead. This is enough, and it is the foundation for successful partnership with the child.

When we are getting to know a child, we will be mostly listening. If they say anything, either with their speech or another modality, we will acknowledge this. We will have to work out which way they prefer us to acknowledge their communication. We may repeat exactly what they say: this is a good way to demonstrate we are listening closely. We won't recast or expand on what they said, as we are showing that we value their language. Some children may feel more comfortable with us nodding or vocalising to acknowledge their communication turn. Some children may like a more enthusiastic vocalisation than others. This is all part of getting to know a child, and honouring their communication preferences.

We talk naturally for at least 50% of the time

We are only consciously modelling language for about 50% of the time. For the rest of the time we are just talking naturally to keep the connection going. We do not want to bombard the child with language modelling. We will make judicious use of silence to allow the child to process and formulate their ideas and their language. If we are talking too much, we will be interrupting their natural flow and not allowing space for processing. This is one of the biggest challenges of this approach, and it is worth regularly videoing sessions so that we can monitor our output compared with the child's. A complete language sample will also show very clearly if our output is exceeding the child's.

For the first few sessions we are listening deeply and valuing the child's natural communication. We acknowledge their communication (spoken and non-verbal) by nodding, vocalising, or repeating back their words or phrases. Once we have gotten to know them, we may drop in some conscious language modelling, and then we will observe the child's response. We are learning about what language the child finds interesting and engaging; we want to provide a memorable and enjoyable soundtrack to this experience.

We might try to work out the musical features of speech that they are drawn to. For example, their preferred pitch-range, using a musical quality to our voice, or a rhythmic quality that matches their actions. We might experiment with funny voices and actions. We might include movement-based songs.

We can model multi-modal communication

If a child is minimally or non-speaking, or if their stage 1 language is highly unintelligible, we might also be using AAC alongside our spoken language modelling (see Chapter 12 for more on this). We will still be thinking about making the soundtrack of this experience interesting and engaging for this child. In our AAC use, we will monitor whether they seem to like whole phrases or sequences of phrases being modelled. We will experiment with digitised voice, recorded speech or a recording from the original sound source.

We might be bringing in written text (see Chapter 13). Our approach is tailored to the child in front of us, and we are endlessly curious about what appeals to them.

At stage 1, GLPs are often unintelligible

At stage 1, GLPs might be unintelligible much of the time. It can be difficult to understand what they are saying. Parents are likely to be the best at working this out. They will have lived through many of the same experiences, and will recognise the soundtrack that the child is trying to recreate, be it a word or phrase a family member has used, a line from a song or a book, or a script from a YouTube clip or a tv programme. Siblings may also be invaluable, since they often consume the same digital media!

Identifying the possible communication intention

If we are not working with a child with their parent in the room with us, we might consider audio or video recording our sessions so that we can later share unintelligible (and intelligible) gestalts with parents for them to try to identify.

We might pick out a word or two, and this may be enough for a parent to identify the source, and then work out the possible communication intention for the child.

There may be some language gestalts, particularly those scripts from tv, movies or YouTube, that even the parent does not recognise. There are some websites that can help us identify particular fragments of tv and movie scripts, or of songs, if we can understand the child's language. At the time of writing these include 'Play Phrase', 'Yarn', 'Subzin', 'QuoDB' and 'Pop Mystic'.

Once we know the source of a gestalt, we need to work out the possible meaning, or communication intention. Where and when the child uses it will give us an indication. Remember that the words are not literal: sometimes a child might have a gestalt like 'welcome to the show!' but for them it means 'I'm really scared and overwhelmed in this situation'.

Single word gestalts

It is possible for a GLP to have picked up a lot of single words. If a parent was advised to use simple language and to model single words, their child may have a lot of single word gestalts. They may look like they are referential, and that they are labelling the 'car', 'dog' and so on.

If the child has not been able to progress to combining these words, despite having the commonly cited 50 single words that ALPs typically need before they start making two-word combinations, then we may be looking at a GLP with 'stuck' single word gestalts.

A GLP who has a lot of 'stuck' single word gestalts may not be using the words referentially in the conventional sense of a word representing a shared meaning. The common shared meaning for the word 'horse' is 'this big animal with a mane and hooves'. But for a GLP, the language gestalt of 'horse' may mean 'remember that time we gave carrots to the thing with big hairy lips and it tickled?' If they are a GLP, then they are likely to be drawn to the 'whole' experience, sensory and emotional resonance included. They are less likely to have been able to extract a semantic definition of 'horse'. This makes it very difficult to progress to word + word combinations.

Listen to the intonation pattern of the single word. Is it always said in the same way? This is a clue that it is a gestalt, and not a conventionally referential word which is ready to be combined with another.

A referential ALP child will sometimes say 'horse' with a falling intonation pattern, as if to say 'it's a horse'. Sometimes they will say 'horse?' with a rising intonation pattern, as if to say 'is it a horse?' There may be some other intonation patterns to express subtleties like 'that's a horse too! Who knew?' or 'I think it's a horse, but can you just confirm this?'

We can't just 'add a word' to a language gestalt

A referential ALP child will quickly move on to word + word combinations using their acquired word 'horsie'. They will soon say 'horsie carrot', 'horsie field', 'horsie naughty', 'dirty horsie', 'there horsie', 'horsie gone' and so on.

A GLP's next stage in language development is to segment the sound-stream into shorter chunks. This can't be done with a single word. We cannot support a stage 1 GLP by 'adding on' to their gestalt. The next step for them is to 'break it down'.

If a language gestalt is a phrase, then the next natural stage for a GLP is to start to break the phrase down into shorter segments, culminating in them knowing where the word boundaries are.

How do we identify if a single word is a 'stuck' gestalt?

- Have we only ever heard this word in isolation? If we have never heard it in combination (in a stage 2 mitigation, in a stage 3 word + word combination or stage 4 early sentence), it's stage 1.

- Is it always said with the same intonation pattern? If so, it is more likely to be being processed as a whole language gestalt: a stage 1 utterance.

What do we do with 'stuck' single words?

Some stage 1 GLPs will have lots of 'stuck' single words because well-intentioned adults have encouraged them to label items: animals, foods, clothes, colours. . . .

We will acknowledge these words when a child says them. We might model a phrase that could become a new gestalt. For example, if a child says, 'aeroplane', we might say, 'flying in the sky', or 'up there!' We're not 'adding on' to their single word in the sense of taking their single word and making it into a two- or three- word phrase, but we are supplying a phrase which relates to their implied communication intention.

Dual processors

There are children who are dual processors and can acquire single referential words alongside language gestalts. These are the children that we likely never see as Speech and Language Therapists, because their use of both analytic and gestalt strategies set them up well for language acquisition. We need more research to understand the relative prevalence of dual processors and GLPs.

From anecdotal evidence, it seems that dual processors go through phases of using analytic strategies more at some stages in their language acquisition, and then using gestalt strategies more, and then integrating the two. For instance a child might acquire lots of single words first, and present like an ALP, but then go through a period of acquiring lots of gestalt phrases. They may then become very fluent mitigators, and then start using their single words in word + word combinations.

We need much more research and parent information about dual processors. In order to support these children we will need to partner with parents to find out what strategies the child is currently using, and support accordingly. If they seem to have moved from ALP single word acquisition to GLP phrases, we would support them like we would a GLP in stage 1. From anecdotal parent evidence, it seems that then there is a fairly rapid progression through the NLA stages.

Encourage everyone to get involved with tracking stage 1 language gestalts

One of the first steps for us as a therapist is to start compiling a list of this child's stage 1 language gestalts. A shared Google document is a great way to do this, because it can then be shared (with the parent's consent) with the parents, any other caregivers and everyone in the child's educational setting.

That way everyone can help to do the detective work to work out what the longer or more nuanced gestalts might mean for this child.

You can see a template for this 'Language Tracker' shared document in the handouts section.

We will note down what the language gestalt is, word for word if possible. If the gestalt has a lot of unclear speech in it, then it is helpful if we can try to transcribe it, or get a sense of the syllable structure, if there are defined syllables. Some gestalts might consist more of open vowels or the intonation pattern. In this case, try to capture a sense of the voice quality, pitch or volume, and any other striking features. Note down when the gestalt is used, and you may begin to see a pattern.

If the child uses AAC or text, or any other communication mode, we will note this in their language tracker. It is possible for a child's language gestalts to be a sequence of Makaton signs or symbols: if the sequence is the same each time, it is likely a gestalt. If it starts to change, it is likely moving into stage 2 mitigation.

A stage 1 gestalt will not have a 'literal' meaning

Stage 1 gestalts are language wholes. That means they will contain everything about the experience for this child, including its sensory qualities and the emotional resonance. It is impossible for us to know exactly the finely nuanced meaning for this child, but we can make a 'good enough' guess with repeated exposure to it, and careful observation.

We can try to gauge the emotion behind the gestalt. We can carefully observe the child's facial expression, level of body tension, their voice quality, volume or rate. Do they seem excited? Delighted? Scared? Worried? The nuances are important.

We can try to see if there are sensory commonalities when they use this gestalt. Does the child always use it when they are looking closely at water in a shower spray, be it from a watering can, the showerhead in the bath or when it is raining?

Some language gestalts are easier than others. A child might sing 'when you feel so mad that you want to roar', a song from Daniel Tiger, when they are frustrated. Some gestalts are more obscure. Longer gestalts are especially challenging, as there are so many potential meanings from a script that is 20 lines long! Listen out for any slower, louder, clearer or emphasised parts, the part which carries a lot of emotion: this is likely to be the part that has the resonance for the child.

We honour the child's language gestalts

Gestalts from songs, tv and film clips can be richly resonant and can be used extremely creatively to express emotional meaning. Adult GLPs tell us that some gestalts are so perfect and beautiful that they would not want to be without them. We can see their point:

• Whatever just happened, blame it on the pig . . . ('Moana')

• Well, bust my buffers! ('Thomas and Friends')

- Dogs like to feel PRETTY! ('Charlie and Lola')

- Good Morning, my fine feathered friends! (Quentin Blake's 'Cockatoos')

We listen intently to all of the child's naturally acquired language, including their longer or more obscure gestalts. We respect these gestalts because this is a GLP's love language. Gestalts will continue to make up an important part of their natural language.

Once we have earned a child's trust, we may also start to think about the communication intention served by longer scripts. We might offer a new phrase that fulfils this communication intention. We might offer a trimmed down version of their stage 1 gestalt, or another phrase that will be mitigable in stage 2.

There is no universal stage 1 phrase checklist

But there are commonly modelled types of phrases. Useful mitigable phrases might start with 'let's', 'we can', 'need to', 'time to', 'got to', 'that's', 'it's' and 'there's'.

We might share the handout 'Some useful phrases to model', found in the handouts section of this book, with parents or teaching staff. We will add a caveat: we always personalise the language we use with a child, depending on their play interests, sensory preferences, preferred activities and so on. This is why it is so important to establish connection and trust first: we are seeing the world through the child's eyes and so we will get to know what lights them up, what shuts them down, the ideas they are likely to want to express, their unique take on the world. . . .

Ultimately we want to be modelling a variety of language. Think about a range of language structures (noun phrases, verb phrases, etc) and a range of communication intentions (sharing ideas, expressing shared joy, describing, protesting, expressing sensory needs, self-advocating, etc). In the handouts section there is a handout called 'Examples of Useful Phrases' that we may share with other adults who are supporting the GLP. This handout is only a starting point: actual children that we work with will provide richer inspiration for more creative and profound thoughts!

Avoid choice-making

Making choices is not an appropriate 'goal' for a GLP. GLPs are not referential until stage 3, so a single symbol choice-board is not helpful. They will be able to show us their interests more effectively by being offered a choice of play experiences. We can then model language like 'this one looks fun' or 'how about painting?' (this is a rhetorical question!)

Avoiding the 'you' pronoun

We avoid modelling phrases beginning with the pronoun 'you'. This pronoun can be problematic for a couple of different reasons. If we narrate what the child is doing (as many of us learnt to do in 'Non-directive therapy') by saying phrases like 'you're pushing the car', a GLP will pick up this whole phrase. They will say 'you're pushing the car'. This is probably more confusing than 'let's push the car'.

Many GLPs have been treated like ALPs. They have been taught phrases like 'I want'. If they have this sort of 'taught language' it will have become a gestalt. If it has been drilled into them, then they will likely slip into it even if they want to access a different phrase beginning with 'I'. For children with a lot of 'I want' phrases, we might model phrases starting with 'need to' and 'got to' rather than 'I need to' and 'I've got to'. For children who have never received PECS or have not been 'taught' phrases, this may not be such a problem.

Avoiding questions

We try to model declarative language. That is, we comment, we observe, we make suggestions, we describe. We don't ask a stage 1 GLP questions, as they will pick up the question as a whole. They will say 'do you want a drink?' when they mean 'I'm thirsty'. They will say 'do you need help?' when they mean 'I need help'. Questions are not the most useful language models for stage 1 GLPs. We model from the child's perspective when we are modelling phrases for requesting.

Rich intonation and musicality

GLPs tend to be highly musical, and many may have perfect pitch. Our more musically inclined colleagues including Corinne Zmoos[1] have observed that GLPs are more likely to take up phrases when they are modelled with intervals of an octave (think 'Somewhere over the rainbow!'), a fifth (think 'Twinkle Twinkle') or a fourth (think 'Here comes the bride'). If that is too complicated, just think 'highly musical' and try to be tuneful and dramatic!

We can also think about the pitch-range that a child uses, and model our language within this pitch range. We know that auditory processing can be an issue for autistic children. The pitch range that they habitually use is likely a range that they can hear or prefer.

Some children may enjoy rhythmic qualities to speech: we might match our rhythm to the communication intention or the meaning of the words. We may employ onomatopoeia (using words that sound like the concept they describe), e.g. 'hop little bunnies, hop hop hop' or using our voice very expressively to match the emotion 'oh! I bumped my head!'

We might also experiment with our voice quality. If a child has a lot of gestalts that come from favourite characters in video clips, think about using funny voices: dopey voices, excited voices, whiny voices, growly voices, outraged voices and so on.

Retraining our ALP brains

Stage 1 GLP language modelling takes practice, particularly as most of us have been taught to model language for Analytic Language Processing. We will probably find that some of this language spills out of us accidentally. As long as we notice this, we are learning. It gets much easier with practice.

Co-regulation and authenticity

GLPs are very sensitive to what is in the room with them, including the energy that we bring. It is very important that we tune into our own regulation so that we do not dysregulate a child by our anxious presence. We may need to check in with ourselves and probe why we are talking too much or trying too hard to engage a child. It is likely that we have ideas about how a therapist should behave or what they should show to a parent.

Experiment with saying less and doing less. We are here to offer calm presence, and to learn from the child, not to have the answers already.

We need to bring our authentic selves to each interaction with a child. If we want them to 'unmask' and communicate naturally, then we also need to be natural, spontaneous and true to ourselves. We are allowed to make mistakes, and we will. We will overstep the mark or misinterpret a child's communication intentions. When this happens, we can be explicit in acknowledging this. When we sing and they don't like it, we can say sorry and try to remember this for the future. When we offer an unwelcome idea, we can pull it back and respect the child's plan. This honesty fosters trust and connection.

Partnering with parents and educators

Parents may know as much, or more, about this approach, compared with us. They certainly know their child better, and spend much more time with them. Parents will ideally talk naturally for at least 50% of the time, and may be consciously modelling for the rest of the time. They too will be prioritising trust and connection, monitoring the child's response to our supports, and adjusting to the child's feedback. If the child is comfortable and engaged and sharing their stage 1 communication, then we are probably getting it right.

For parents and educators who have been trained in analytic language development approaches, or who use techniques to elicit or prompt language, we will need to address this directly and provide information to explain our approach. There are handouts on the Communication Development Center, including the shorter 'NLA International Handout' translated into an ever increasing range of languages, and the longer 'Natural Language Acquisition Guide'. There is also an 'Introduction to GLP' handout in the handouts section of this book.

As we know, different people like to learn in different ways. There are also introduction webinars available on the Communication Development Center, Natural Communication and Meaningful Speech websites.

For educators especially, it can be helpful to talk about declarative language and avoiding questions at this stage. Typical supports that are recommended on EHCP reports (or other 'programmes' or provision plans) may need to be revised. For example, choice-making with single words or symbols, Now-and-Next boards, the introduction of core words through a communication board. These can be tweaked, replacing single words with phrases, but we also want to consider the individual child. Many of these 'supports' imply that a child has limited understanding of language and so needs visual support in order to understand. We can no longer assume that this is the case. GLP children are likely to be able to participate and understand when we partner them and see the world through their eyes, try to understand their communication intentions and model relevant and appealing language, and are honest and genuine when we don't get it, or get things wrong.

Summary of stage 1 supports

- Establish trust and connection with a child. Without this, our language is unlikely to resonate.

- Keep communication going by doing 'just enough' to keep the connection going. If we notice that we are doing too much, we pull back, allowing the child to lead again.

- Offer silence and space so that the child can think and process.

- Provide opportunities for playful movement and unrestricted access to regulatory supports.

- Monitor our own regulation. When we are 'just playing' and offering language we need to remind ourselves that 'we are enough' and that we are doing enough, especially when other adults are observing our sessions.

- Show the child that we are authentic in our interactions. If we make a mistake, we acknowledge it.

- Value and validate all of the child's communication, including their multi-modal communication, in whatever form these take (video clips, recited scripts, gestures, signs, action routines, AAC messages and so on).

- Partner with parents to find the source of language gestalts. Think about what these gestalts might mean for the child and what communication intention they fulfil.

- Talk naturally at least 50% of the time.

- Once trust and connection is established, offer possible language to match the child's communication intentions.

- Use language that is appealing to the child. This may take time to work out!

- Experiment with rich intonation and monitoring the child's response.

- Experiment with songs to match a communication intention, or to accompany particular routines, e.g. a tidy-up song, a getting dressed song.

- Experiment with other musical qualities that the child might be drawn to: the pitch-range that the child is attracted to, rhythmic qualities, funny voices. . . .

- Provide multi-modal language modelling for minimally speaking, non-speaking or highly unintelligible GLPs. We might provide paper-based or iPad-based AAC. We may write down our spoken language.

- Take regular language samples to track a child's language acquisition.

- Respect the time a child needs to take in order to fully explore stage 1 language before they begin to mitigate and use stage 2 language. We might try a mitigation after acknowledging their stage 1 gestalt, but if they are not responding to this, we go back to acknowledging their gestalt without trying to change it. We do not want to lose their trust by trying to rush them through the stages.

How we track progress in stage 1

We will use our language tracker and language samples to look at the gestalts a child has acquired, across modalities (e.g. spoken language, paper-based AAC, iPad-based AAC). We are looking at the variety in the communication intentions. We are looking at the variety in language structures, as this will support variety in stage 2. If we notice gaps, we might think about how to best provide language models that will be appealing for this child. We might compile a table like Table 5.2 (there is a template for this, 'Communication Intentions Inventory', in the handouts section):

Table 5.2 Communication Intentions Inventory

Communication intention	Examples
Talking about special interests and enthusiasms	Daniel: eyes, nose, mouth, ears, stripes, whiskers! (requesting we draw these) Run away! (requesting a game where we hide) Red, orange, yellow, green, blue, purple, brown (requesting colours of paint)
Sharing ideas	It's a dinosaur Run away! Not enough! There you are
Expressing shared joy; shared play routines	Surprise! Come on! Ok, George, open your eyes! I want to turn around
Describing objects, people or activities	All the colours Here it is Very tall! So big!
Protesting	Go away! Oh no! Don't do that! No thank you
Transitioning	Tidy up Coat, ready to go Shoes on

Goals for a stage 1 GLP

This is *Natural* Language Acquisition. As such, we cannot predict what language will be taken up. SCRUFFY goals are more appropriate than SMART goals (for more explanation of SCRUFFY goals, see my first book, *Who's Afraid of AAC?*). SCRUFFY goals allow wiggle room. We don't specify exactly which words or phrases will be acquired, but we describe the broad type of language that the child is likely to acquire.

We specify in the goal that the child is well-regulated. There is more on sensory regulation in Chapter 10. We also specify that the activity is child-led and self-chosen, and that the communication partner has knowledge of NLA. That way the communication that is being 'measured' in a goal is natural communication and not prompted by an adult.

For example, an early stage 1 goal might be:

> **With unlimited access to her chosen regulatory supports and in a self-chosen activity with a communication partner who has knowledge of Natural Language Acquisition (NLA), Rose will spontaneously use her language gestalts to express a range of communication intentions. Rose might express her language gestalts using spoken language (mouth words) or using AAC.**

A later stage 1 goal might be:

> **With unlimited access to her chosen regulatory supports and in a self-chosen activity with a communication partner who has knowledge of Natural Language Acquisition (NLA), Rose will acquire 5–10 new language gestalts to express a range of communication intentions.**

Case study: Rose

Rose first came to see me when she was 5 years old. She already had a diagnosis of autism. She was in preschool, but was about to transition into reception class at her local primary school. Becky, her mum, had delayed this by a year, feeling that Rose would benefit from more time in her familiar preschool setting.

Rose came with her mum into my therapy room looking a little wary and unsure. I chatted to Becky whilst Rose settled into exploring toys. I gave Rose space and silence.

As Rose played, she began to vocalise very quietly. It was something between humming, and open vowels, and then occasionally, very quietly, some strings of syllables which sounded like a possible script. I asked Becky if Rose liked watching video clips and if she every recited the scripts. Becky said that Rose loved Peppa Pig and Daniel Tiger. Becky had not ever thought about whether Rose was reciting the scripts. Maybe she was.

At this stage, I was mostly being very quiet, but I did catch a string of consonants that I could copy back. I had noticed the same string a couple of times within a longer script, and this string was slightly louder and more emphatic. I attempted to repeat it.

Rose stopped what she was doing and looked straight at me. She happens to have the most piercing blue eyes, and this was quite a moment. I smiled, and she continued to hold my gaze. She looked away, and then went back to what she was doing. I got quiet again and just listened. Rose resumed her very quiet vocalisations, and I strained my ears to listen in.

About mid-way through our session, Rose gravitated towards the musical instruments. By now she appeared quite comfortable with my presence. I moved a little closer and I showed her how each musical instrument made a noise. I played them quietly, as I was not sure about Rose's auditory sensitivities. Rose reached for the drumsticks and banged them on the drum. She clearly enjoyed this, and so I sang, 'I like to bang on the drum drum drum!' matching Rose's drum beats. I tried to be as musical and richly intonational as possible. Rose looked straight at me. We repeated this, and Rose smiled. To my utter delight, Rose joined in with this: she was using the same phrase with the same intonation pattern. The words 'bang' and 'drum' were easy to hear within the intonational pattern.

Towards the end of the session, Rose moved to her mum and climbed on her lap. She started to initiate a game that they often played, 'I see you!' Rose would move Becky's hands, so that they covered Becky's eyes, and then she would pull them open and Becky would say, 'I see you!' Rose would then join in and say, 'I see you!' at the same time.

At the end of our session, I talked to Becky about how I was going to assume that Rose is a GLP. I gave a handout with basic information about this.

We talked about really listening in to Rose's super quiet vocalisations, because I suspected that these were scripts from her favourite tv shows. I got Becky's permission to start a shared document for logging Rose's language. We could already add 'I see you!' to this document.

By the following session, Becky had added a few more phrases and some single words to the shared document. They included 'Surprise!' and 'Stop!' which were two games that Rose loved to play with her parents. Becky had also noticed that Rose did seem to be repeating back scripts from 'Peppa Pig' and 'Daniel Tiger', but they were very quiet and very indistinct at the moment.

By the time Rose started her new school, she was vocalising throughout our sessions together. Rose loved musical instruments and singing, and she loved to build towers with some wooden threading beads. Our shared document of Rose's language had grown to three pages long. It consisted of fragments of scripts that we could just make out, like 'open your eyes, George!' from Peppa Pig, her favourite songs, like 'When you feel so mad' from Daniel Tiger, some new phrases like 'there you go' and 'I don't want to' and a few single words like 'strawberry' and 'delicious'.

I went to visit Rose in her new class. Although I had planned to take her out of class and work with her and a teaching assistant in a space where we could move around and possibly use some gym equipment, Rose's TA explained that Rose was reluctant to leave her classroom at the moment. We tried to tempt her with her favourite set of threading beads, but Rose took these back to the quiet corner of the classroom. We agreed that I should see Rose in the classroom.

This turned out to work really well. Rose explored the home corner and then the painting corner. I could listen in to her language gestalts and acknowledge them quietly, and repeat back fragments that I heard. I could also add the odd new phrase to keep the conversation going: 'baby needs her nappy changed', and 'sh! She's sleeping'.

The teaching staff identified that they could replace questions with phrases like 'let's wash hands'. They also had access to the shared document and could add any new language that they heard, and Rose's likely communication intention when she used it.

Over the next few weeks, teaching staff got to know Rose. They learnt that there were recurring themes in her play that they could build on. For example, she enjoyed role-playing 'Dr Rose' using a stethoscope and notepad. She liked a rainbow construction puzzle, and this led to drawing and painting rainbows. She loved building towers, and was making increasingly complex constructions. Staff were open to Rose's ideas, and took videos and photos to share with her parents.

Rose also had access to a GLP-friendly communication book. In addition to her own language gestalts, it had some new phrases, organised into communication intentions like: expressing ideas, shared joy, protesting, transitions, sensory needs and self-advocacy. Adults modelled these without expectation, as well as using natural language for at least 50% of the time. Rose often looked at the communication book when phrases were modelled, and sometimes she took the adult's finger to a phrase to request that they say it for her. She picked up a few new gestalts in this way, including 'go away' and 'I don't like it'.

By now Rose was very much recognised as a communicator, including by her peers, and she was enjoying some special friendships with a couple of other children. Her teacher told me at the end of her third term at school 'Rose understands everything. And she can communicate pretty effectively. We just need to listen'.

Note

1 At Crescendo Communication: crescendocommunication.com

Chapter 6

Stage 2

Mitigations

Whilst stage 1 is deeply meaningful, often emotionally charged and profound in its personal significance for this child, stage 2 becomes more easily understood by a communication partner. It is that bit more transparent, and so even less familiar communication partners are likely to follow a child's intended meaning. Children are more obviously sharing their ideas, thoughts and feelings. Our role continues to be to accompany them, receive their communication, and show that we 'get it'.

Revision: the six stages of Natural Language Acquisition

Let's look at stage 2 in the context of its previous and future stages, in Table 6.1:

Table 6.1 The six stages of Natural Language Acquisition

		Examples
Stage 1	Language gestalts (wholes, scripts, songs, language soundtracks from experiences)	Zoom zoom zoom, we're going to the moon! It's a dinosaur!
Stage 2	Mitigations: a) Shortening long gestalts b) Dividing them into chunks c) Recombining different chunks	We're going to the moon! We're going! We're going to the shops! It's an octopus!
Stage 3	Isolated single words Word + word combinations of referential single words	dinosaur; rocket dinosaur . . . big; rocket . . . up
Stage 4	Original phrases and beginning sentences	We got dinosaur Put rocket up there
Stage 5	Original sentences with more complex grammar	I can get the dinosaurs I don't want to put my shoes on
Stage 6	Original sentences culminating in a complete grammar system	Who could have taken the dinosaurs? I've been looking for my shoes

DOI: 10.4324/9781032717029-6

How do we know when a child is moving into stage 2?

The child will naturally move into stage 2 when they have enough language material in stage 1. They will have variety in terms of phrase structure, and in terms of communication intentions. The length of time a child spends in stage 1 will vary: this process is natural to them and can't be hurried. Their interests, inclinations and individual processing will determine their chosen gestalts. They will have a unique collection of gestalts which will provide unique possibilities to mitigation.

There are a few ways in which a gestalt might be 'mitigated':

- A long gestalt might be 'trimmed down'. For example, the lines from 'The Highway Rat' might be trimmed from 'The Highway Rat was a baddie, The Highway Rat was a beast. He took what he wanted and ate what he took. His life was one long feast'. This might be trimmed down to 'The Highway Rat was a baddie, the Highway Rat was a beast'.

- This trimming process might happen several times with long gestalts, with the chunks getting shorter and shorter. In the previous example, we might have 'the Highway Rat was a beast' and 'he took what he wanted'.

- Mitigations may get trimmed down into single word mitigations. These single words will be coded as stage 2 because we know they originally came from a gestalt. Only when we hear them being used referentially as a single word and also in a novel word + word combination will we score this word as a stage 3.

- The original gestalt might be made into a 'frame-and-slot' with new material being slotted into the original gestalt. Using the previous example, we might get 'the Highway Rat was . . . hungry' or 'The Highway Rat was . . . gone'.

- There might be a mix-and-matching of gestalts where different chunks can be recombined in new ways. For example, 'I need to move' and 'time to go' might be combined into 'I need . . . to go' or 'time . . . to move'. There are likely to be grammatical discrepancies: these chunks will not always sit perfectly from a grammatical point of view. For example, we might hear 'I need . . . a mummy' or 'time to . . . one long feast'. This is a good sign, though. It shows that the child is actively playing with language and seeing what it can do.

- A gestalt may be mitigated (changed) with a new intonation pattern. The words may be the same, but it is clear that the intention has changed: a new nuance of meaning is being conveyed. This is another indication that the child is appreciating the flexibility of their language: they can modulate meaning by slightly altering pitch, rhythm, volume, melodic intonation.

Children are naturally exposed to 'frame-and-slot' mitigations in stories and songs. For example, 'Brown bear, brown bear, what do you see? I see a . . . (blue horse;

yellow duck) looking at me', or 'This is the way we . . . (wash our hands; brush our hair)'. We can sing these songs and tell these stories if a child is interested in them. They will provide natural material for mitigation. However we don't want to force stage 2, and we wouldn't prompt a child to swop in a new chunk; we would just model it in a fun game.

Stage 2 is momentous

Stage 2 opens up huge potential variety in terms of language content and structure, but also in terms of communication intentions. Stage 1 language was highly meaningful for the child, but stage 2 is more obviously meaningful and transparent for a wider range of communication partners. The child's intentionality is clear to everyone, and this is powerful for the child, as they are widely viewed as communicatively competent. The child can now potentially experience communication success with a wider range of people, in a wider range of situations, and so their language exposure increases.

A child can express an awful lot at this stage, and for many children or adults, stage 2 might be a stopping-off point. There are many autistic adults who describe their language as being made up of mix-and-match chunks. Stage 2 language offers infinite possibilities in mix-and-matching language chunks. It may be an onerous process for a GLP to trawl through their ever expanding collection of stage 1 and stage 2 language in order to find the right chunks, but it is possible to be an articulate communicator using this process. Of course, there are benefits to going on through the later stages of NLA and having the ultimate flexibility of a complete grammar system, but we so also need to acknowledge the incredible variety and complexity that can be expressed using stage 2 language.

The importance of language samples

As we partner a child through this process, our language samples will guide us. We will only be able to recognise a stage 2 mitigation if we know their stage 1 language. We will be familiar with the intonation pattern and vocal features of a particular gestalt, and so we will notice when it is trimmed down or mix-and-matched.

This is where it is helpful to audio or video record language samples. From a one-time live listening, we might think we mis-heard. Being able to listen back later gives us assurance that we did indeed hear a mitigation.

Speech is not the only communication mode. If a child's gestalts are in signs or symbols, or in actions, or in text, then their mitigations will also likely take this mode.

If language samples are showing us that a child has been in stage 1 for a long time with no sign of mitigation, we will want to think about the variety in their stage 1 language. Questions we might ask ourselves include:

- Is the language that we are modelling appealing to them? We might consider our pitch-range, the melodic or rhythmic qualities that they are drawn to, the voice qualities that they like, the media they are drawn to, their preferred communication modes. . . .

- Are the experiences that we are providing lighting them up? Do we need to think about their sensory preferences, their movement needs, their play preferences, their enthusiasms?

- Are they well-regulated when we are modelling language? For them to be receptive to our modelling they need to be in a good place. Could we be unintentionally dysregulating them in some way?

- What communicative intentions are they currently expressing? Is there sufficient variety? Do they need more language around protesting, self-advocating, meeting their regulation needs? What communication intentions would be powerful or profound for them?

The importance of variety

As a child explores stage 2, we will look in their language samples for variety. We can increase the likely variety by providing for a range of experiences. In stage 1 we were providing memorable, engaging experiences for which a child might retain the soundtrack. In stage 2 we are continuing to provide novel experiences, so that the child can continue to add to their widening repertoire of language experiences. We might think about providing experiences that offer access to new vocabulary, new phrase structures, new communication intentions. If we notice in repeated language samples that the child is only mitigating around a few 'frame-and-slot' structures, we may want to model more stage 1 phrases.

We can offer a wide range of play experiences, but we don't need to push this. We can gently offer similar toys or games to those that we know the child enjoys. If they love dinosaurs, they might also like wild animals. If they love throwing balls, they might like balloons or bean-bags. If they love playdough, they might like kinetic sand or cornflour. Each new experience offers new possibilities.

When a child is in stage 2 more communication partners will see them as competent, and so there is naturally more potential for language variety. Different communication partners will introduce different language structures. New language gestalts are likely to be acquired, and this will add to the mix for stage 2 explorations.

When do we intentionally model stage 2 language?

We will continue to use natural language for at least 50% of the time. Just like in stage 1, our primary purpose (as it is throughout the NLA journey) is to keep the connection alive. We are carefully and sensitively observing what a child is into right now, and joining them in this experience.

That being said, when we are intentionally modelling language, there will be a subtle shift in our language modelling when our language samples show that a child is starting to mitigate. We might take a phrase that they have already mitigated and add another variation. For example, if they have sung 'I see triceratops' and then 'I see tyrannosaurus' in the next verse, we might model 'I see brontosaurus'. If they say, 'up up up the stairs' and then 'down down down the stairs', we might model 'up up up the ramp' and 'down down down the ramp'.

Songs and stories are very helpful for mitigation. Songs such as 'This is the way we . . .', 'If you're happy and you know it . . .', 'The wheels on the bus . . .' and 'Old Macdonald' offer natural opportunities for mitigation. Stories with repeated refrains and slight variations, such as *Dear Zoo*, *Brown Bear, Brown Bear*, *We're Going on a Bear Hunt* and *Ketchup on Your Cornflakes* all demonstrate mitigation.

Offering a range of experiences through play and movement will naturally inspire opportunities for mitigation. If a child has gestalts for expressing joy, expressing sensory preferences, protesting, self-advocating and so on, then varying the activity will naturally provide material for mitigation. If they have a gestalt like 'jumping is fun!' or 'need to bounce', then there are rich pickings for natural mitigation.

But we don't want to force the issue. The best way to model is to take what the child is doing already and go with the flow. This is a partnership, and we want the child to be leading us, rather than the other way around. We will look at how they are naturally mitigating. They may not need much conscious effort from us if they are mitigating freely in a variety of contexts, with different communication partners and with different communication intentions. If they are only mitigating a limited number of gestalts or limited communication intentions, then we might want to revisit their stage 1 language and provide for more variety.

There is no universal stage 1 or stage 2 checklist

Remember that there is no universal stage 1 phrase checklist, and so there will be no stage 2 checklist. The child will develop their own unique repertoire. This is the beauty of NLA for a Speech and Language Therapist. No one child's journey will ever the same as another child's. It is endlessly fascinating, endlessly creative.

Don't force progression: this is *Natural* Language Acquisition

It is tempting to want to fast-track this process. We desperately want to hear the child create their first stage 2 language.

We know from approaches such as ABA and PECS that we can 'elicit' language from a GLP. We can teach them to say phrases such as 'I want biscuit' and 'I want pizza'. But we also know that this taught language does not necessarily translate into self-generated language. It often just leads to 'prompt dependency'.

The child leads us into their stage 2, and through their stage 2. We wait for their first mitigations, and then we start modelling a few more. Not the other way around.

Variety in stage 2

Natural Language Acquisition is allowing the child to spend enough time in each stage for the child to explore all the possibilities. We continue to model potential gestalts. This provides more language variety that will support subsequent NLA stages.

The process can appear slow, and may take months, but this is language acquisition, and it does take time. A child may only mitigate two different stage 1 gestalts for a while. Then one or two more may appear. There may be a speeding up of mitigations as the child becomes more firmly established in stage 2. Access to a variety of playful experiences with different communication partners is likely to provide rich opportunities for mitigation.

Stage 2 is not referential . . . yet

GLPs are not referential yet, but their stage 2 'frames-and-slots' will likely lead them there. Phrases like 'it's an elephant!' and 'it's a giraffe!' will help them move towards isolating the words 'elephant' and 'giraffe'.

Stage 2 'grammar'

Stage 2 GLPs may be using a range of verb tenses, plurals and contractions. But they have not processed these as self-generated original grammar yet. They have 'lifted' that chunk of language wholesale, without actively analysing the grammatical constructions within it.

For example, Alex, who is featured in the case study in Chapter 8, used the language chunk 'so they all rolled over' in his stage 2 language. He had lifted this from the song 'There were 10 in the bed'. He was not yet actively processing that the pronoun 'they' is plural, that past tense regular verbs have an '-ed' ending or that the conjunction 'so' is used to explain an idea earlier in the sentence. That will be for later stages.

For this reason, stage 2 language can sometimes sound a bit 'clunky' and mismatched. The child doesn't yet know which aspects of the language chunk relates to which vocabulary concept, or which part of grammar can be manipulated to modulate meaning. So they might 'mix-and-match' language chunks a little bit oddly, to our ears. For example, 'this one . . . all rolled over' to express that the car fell off the track, or 'can't touch it . . . your shoe' to express that they've hurt their toe.

Keep focusing on the communication intentions of the child

The child will continue to acquire stage 1 language gestalts as they move through later stages of NLA. Gestalts are their first language. We always acknowledge their natural language, even as we are still trying to work out the significance of it. There may be themes in the child's play that help us work out the deeper meaning of their gestalts, and then we are better qualified to provide appropriate language to build on their intentions. Videoing sessions and taking language samples will help us to reflect on the child's communication intentions in context. We will continue to work in partnership with parents, so that we keep abreast of the child's current interests, play, media choices, communication intentions and modes of communication.

Summary of stage 2 supports

There is a high degree of overlap between these supports and those from stage 1. This is because stages are a somewhat artificial construction: they are simply a guide for us. The foundational principles are the same throughout Natural Language Acquisition; we just tweak some of the supports as a child moves through the stages.

- Prioritise trust and connection with a child. We cannot rush the process, and we have to move at their pace.

- Keep communication going by doing 'just enough' to keep the connection going.

- Offer silence and space so that the child can think and process language.

- Provide opportunities for playful movement and unrestricted access to regulatory supports.

- Monitor our own regulation, and take steps to address this if needed.

- Continue to show our authentic selves. If we make a mistake, we acknowledge it.

- Value and validate all of the child's communication, including their gestalts and mitigations.

- Partner with parents to interpret non-literal gestalts and recognise mitigations.

- Talk naturally at least 50% of the time.

- Take a child's natural mitigations and offer more options. We're not bombarding them; we're scattering a few here and there.

- When offering mitigations, we keep the intonational curve as close to their gestalt or mitigation as possible. This helps them make the connection that the language has been 'remixed'.

- Take regular language samples to track a child's language acquisition.

- Offer additional language where a child needs greater variety in their stage 1 or stage 2 language.

- Provide novel experiences for the child: different toys, different books, different play situations . . . these will add to the variety in mitigations.

- Offer opportunities for the child to communicate with new people if their intelligibility is clearer: this will provide even more language variety.

How we track progress in stage 2

Our language samples are really crucial for tracking progress over weeks and months. They allow us to spot any mitigations from stage 1 gestalts. In our written reports, we might show this in a table like the one shown in Table 6.2:

Table 6.2 Examples of mitigations for a specific child

Stage 1 gestalt	Stage 2 mitigations
What a beautiful day. We're not scared.	We're not scared. We're not finished.
Give me your sweets and your lollies, Give me your toffees and chews	Give me your . . . that one!
It's a rainbow! Red, orange, yellow, green, blue, indigo, violet	Rainbow! Red Orange

(Continued)

Stage 1 gestalt	Stage 2 mitigations
Old Macdonald had a farm, ee-ay-ee-ay-oh. And on that farm he had a pig . . .	Ee-ay-ee-ay-oh And on that farm he had a horse . . . pig horse
There were 10 in the bed and the little one said 'Roll over, roll over'	Roll over!
Where are you, aeroplane?	Where are you, dinosaur? Where are you red piece?

Goals for a stage 2 GLP

Just like in stage 1, we write a goal around the broad type of language that the child might acquire, rather than specific mitigations. We might focus on the range of communication intentions. We might specify an increase in the percentage of stage 2 utterances, e.g. an increase from 25% to 50% of a total language sample. We will base this goal on our videoed sessions and language samples so that it is relevant for this particular child.

We continue to specify in the goal that the child is well-regulated, that the activity is child-led and that the communication partner has knowledge of NLA.

A stage 2 goal might be written as:

> ***With unlimited access to her chosen regulatory supports and in a self-chosen activity with a communication partner who has knowledge of Natural Language Acquisition (NLA), Shanti will trim down and remix her language gestalts in order to express new ideas.***

Or:

> ***With unlimited access to her chosen regulatory supports and in a self-chosen activity with a communication partner who has knowledge of Natural Language Acquisition (NLA), Shanti will produce mitigated gestalts across a range of communication intentions, e.g. protesting, self-advocating.***

From language samples, we may feel that even though a child has language from later stages they would still benefit from greater diversity in stage 2, and we might write a goal such as:

> ***With unlimited access to her chosen regulatory supports and in a self-chosen activity with a communication partner who has knowledge of Natural Language Acquisition (NLA), Shanti will use a rich mixture of language across the NLA stages, along with new stage 2 language.***

Case study: Shanti

Shanti was identified as a GLP by her preschool, as they had worked with another child who was also a GLP. They had noted that Shanti used phrases from books and lines from songs in particular contexts. For example, 'All was quiet in the deep dark woods' when she needed to be alone, and 'give me your buns and your biscuits, give me your chocolate eclairs!' when another child took a toy that she was playing with. She loved singing songs, which was a regular part of the preschool session. Shanti's keyworker sought advice from me as I was providing consultative services to their school. Shanti's keyworker did not feel confident about discussing Natural Language Acquisition with Shanti's parents and so arranged for me to meet with them.

Preschool had also made some observations that were indicating that Shanti may be autistic. Shanti's parents had not previously raised anything with them about this.

I discussed the two typical pathways into language acquisition: Analytic and Gestalt Language Processing. Shanti's parents recognised her gestalt processing, and gave some examples of this. For example, Shanti liked to bring in the milk in the morning, and was confused if the delivery had not arrived on time. She had some scripts from 'Hey Duggee' which included actions of jumping up and down and gesticulating.

I talked about the association between GLP and autism. I used strengths-based language when I talked about autism, and explained that the common understanding of autism is not particularly accurate, often focusing on deficits rather than strengths. I listed some of the strengths that Shanti was showing, being skilled already at recognising numbers and letters and remembering whole chunks of complex language. I stressed that autism is very common, and that autistic children are educated in mainstream schools, can be highly educated professionals and grow up to have families and friendship networks.

Shanti's parents were both concerned and engaged. I explained that we know how to support autistic children and GLPs. Shanti's language appeared to be developing naturally along the predictable pattern of Natural Language Acquisition.

From a language sample taken in preschool, it appeared that Shanti was entering stage 2. She was swopping words into different songs, like 'Old Macdonald' and 'This is the way we . . .' There were examples of mitigated phrases: the 'can't go over it, can't go under it, we'll have to go through it' was being reduced to 'we'll have to go through it' and also 'we'll have to go outside and play'.

I presented Shanti's parents with some options, including signposting to relevant websites for more information on NLA. I showed them the NLA handouts from the Communication Development Center website, and suggested that they might watch a couple of videos on the site. Shanti's family were bilingual and so I encouraged them to speak naturally in the languages of their choosing, and offer Shanti access to stories, songs and media in both languages.

We discussed the pros and cons of seeking an autism diagnosis. Shanti's parents were concerned that labelling their daughter might lead to people underestimating her abilities. They were worried about their wider family and network of friends, and how to explain Shanti's needs to them.

We agreed to follow this discussion with a video consultation the following week.

In the meantime, preschool staff were advised to talk naturally with Shanti, responding positively to all of her natural language. They had the NLA handout which suggests relevant supports like 'take the time to see what the child is doing; watch and listen, and provide plenty of silence' and 'comment on what you and the child is doing'.

At the video consultation a week later, Shanti's parents said that they had done a 'deep dive' into GLP and autism. They were not ready to pursue a formal diagnosis of autism, but they had read enough about GLP to recognise that this was the way their daughter was acquiring language. They had read a couple of handouts and these were now stuck to their fridge as a reminder of the supports they could provide for Shanti. We agreed that as both preschool and they were now clear on how to model language, we would check in with one another in four weeks. Preschool would take a video recording to show me at my next consultation visit with them, so that we could track Shanti's language.

The video recording showed that Shanti's stage 2 mitigations were continuing to flourish. She was shown playing with magnetic letters, saying 'it's a letter h for horse. It's a letter e for elephant'. She was shown in the home corner pretending to bake cakes, and she was saying, 'we must add butter' and 'we must stir it'. Her keyworker modelled 'yes, and we must wait for the cake to bake'. Shanti was continuing to acquire stage 1 gestalts too. She had more gestalts for protesting, including 'I will not ever never eat a tomato' (from 'Charlie and Lola') which she used to reject play activities, as well as food.

Two months later Shanti's parents asked preschool how they might go about seeking a diagnosis of autism. They had a family friend who had just had a diagnosis as an adult. They had had long discussions about the benefits of understanding a child's needs, especially from a sensory point of view. Shanti's parents were noticing that Shanti needed outdoor time each day, and needed 'rough-and-tumble' time before bed in order to settle. She had had a big meltdown with her grandparents when they had stopped her from bouncing on the trampoline. Her grandparents had felt that she was being defiant, and Shanti's dad was upset that they had not shown more empathy towards Shanti. Sensory sensitivities might also explain some food preferences. The family were no longer insisting that Shanti ate the same way as they did. She was allowed to eat different foods separately, and she had 'safe' foods available if she rejected the cooked family meal.

I continued to check in with preschool, and observed Shanti another month later. Her mitigations were flowing freely. She was mix-and-matching phrases easily, including 'there's the . . .', 'here's a . . .', 'we've got . . .', 'it's not . . .', 'I will not ever . . .' and 'now it's time for . . .' She was regularly commenting on what she and other children were doing, for example 'Shanti's bouncing on the trampoline' and 'Maisie's jumping on the trampoline'. She loved playing 'Simon Says', calling out the actions and either including or leaving out the 'Simon Says' part. Preschool had been modelling 'I don't like it' so that Shanti had a choice of phrases for protesting, and Shanti had almost instantly mitigated this phrase to 'I don't like it wet sleeve' and 'I don't like it sit there now'.

Preschool also observed that Shanti was beginning to isolate some single words. On my request they took a language sample, which I scored, asking for their input where needed, as I was not familiar with all of Shanti's stage 2 mitigations. Fifty percent of Shanti's utterances were stage 2, with a range of communication intentions. It was also clear from the language sample that Shanti was naturally entering stage 3.

I agreed with preschool and Shanti's parents that it would be good to schedule another video consultation. Since Shanti's language had so far developed very easily with a consultative model of SLT input, we planned for this to continue. By this point Shanti's parents were members of an online community of GLP parents. They felt comfortable asking questions, and often had the answers already: they just needed confirmation and affirmation that they were on the right track.

Chapter 7

Stage 3
Referential single words

Stage 3 marks a momentous step, as the child becomes referential in the conventional sense of being able to point to something and know that we have a single word for the single concept. They have been in a process of whittling down longer gestalts and mitigations until words have been isolated. They recognise word boundaries: the spaces between words that separate out one word's meaning from another word's meaning. They are now in the process of separating out these individual concepts: nouns, attributes, locations . . . and are able to contemplate each word in turn and examine its meaning.

We are here to observe this, and perhaps play with them, looking at each concept in turn, sometimes combining two concepts, and exploring how two concepts can relate to one another to express a variety of different meanings.

Revision: the six stages of Natural Language Acquisition

Let's look at the momentous stage 3 in the context of its previous and future stages (Table 7.1):

Table 7.1 The six stages of Natural Language Acquisition

		Examples
Stage 1	Language gestalts (wholes, scripts, songs, language soundtracks from experiences)	Zoom zoom zoom, we're going to the moon! It's a dinosaur!
Stage 2	Mitigations: a) Shortening long gestalts b) Dividing them into chunks c) Recombining different chunks	We're going to the moon! We're going! We're going to the shops! It's an octopus!

(Continued)

DOI: 10.4324/9781032717029-7

		Examples
Stage 3	Isolated single words Word + word combinations of referential single words	dinosaur; rocket dinosaur . . . big; rocket . . . up
Stage 4	Original phrases and beginning sentences	We got dinosaur Put rocket up there
Stage 5	Original sentences with more complex grammar	I can get the dinosaurs I don't want to put my shoes on
Stage 6	Original sentences culminating in a complete grammar system	Who could have taken the dinosaurs? I've been looking for my shoes

How do we know when a child is moving into stage 3?

As hinted at already, this stage can strike us as sounding very different. A child who has been fluent and melodic in stages 1 and 2 may announce their stage 3 with an apparent reduction in their language output. It may seem as though they have slowed down. We may be lucky enough to witness their first stage 3 utterance. We may note an oddly flat tone, with a large gap between two words.

For some children, particularly younger children, we may not see an obvious shift into single words, but more a whittling down of mitigations. The mitigations get shorter and shorter, and sometimes a mitigation happens to be a single word. We know that they have entered stage 3 when they are able to create new word + word combinations with their newly isolated single words. The child has never done this 'from-the-bottom-up' construction before; it has always been 'from-the-top-down': a longer phrase that they have trimmed down. Now they are taking a single word, and adding another, and constructing from the bottom up: an analytic strategy.

Stage 3 offers the opportunity for a vocabulary explosion. The pathways for learning new words may become more automatic. If the child has been freely mitigating, then perhaps they have now analysed enough frames-and-slots in order to recognise where single words can slot in and out. Therefore we may see greater flexibility in stage 2 alongside entry into stage 3. We may also see a seemingly simultaneous entry into stage 4, with not only stage 3 word + word combinations, but three- and four-word combinations of newly isolated words. For stage 3 especially, there is likely to be a rich mixture of language across multiple stages simultaneously.

Stage 3 may need special attention for older GLPs

For a few GLPs, this stage may happen in their head. Older GLPs might be only too aware that this stage looks like language regression. Their processing may not be apparent in language samples, but subsequent entry into stage 4 implies it has happened. Some adult GLPs have told us that they did not reveal their stage 3 language because they knew that those around them would be alarmed.

But some older GLPs will be delighted with this stage. For the first time they can enjoy referencing games: pointing, showing, checking that we share the same word for a concept, matching two items that share the same name, comparing two items that are similar or different. This stage can be a lot of fun.

For one parent, the dad of Alex, who is featured in the case study in the following chapter, this stage was a real bonding experience for father and son. Alex's dad felt that this stage removed the pressure of perfection. They learnt together how almost everything in the immediate environment can be expressed using word + word combinations. They could look around the room or go on a walk and enjoy combinations like 'sky . . . blue', 'big . . . sky', 'sun . . . warm', 'sun . . . face'. It was a joint venture for them: something that either of them could initiate, knowing that the other person would always respond.

For older children, we may need to partner them in this stage for a while. We may need to ensure that we are exploring the stage fully – the many semantic relationships that are possible in pre-grammar two-word combinations – so that the child is fully equipped for grammar in stage 4.

What are the signs that a child has arrived at stage 3?

- They begin to refer to particular entities and concepts independently by pointing, looking, slowing down and examining them.

- They have access to a good number of stage 2 mitigations. They have variety of vocabulary, phrase types and communication intentions in these mitigations.

- They are starting to use single words referentially, and these same single words are being used in word + word combinations, initiated by the child.

Why couldn't we have started our language modelling at this stage?

We couldn't have started here for a Gestalt Language Processor because their natural strategy is to start with a whole and then break it down into its component words (top-down processing). Single words can't be broken down to create new word + word combinations. Analytic language processors' natural strategy is to start with a single word and then build it up adding word + word (bottom-up processing). This doesn't work for a GLP, no matter how much we model it. Until they have gone through stage 1 phrase-based gestalts and broken them down into stage 2 shorter-phrase mitigations through to isolated word mitigations, they will not be able to treat a single word as a building block for novel phrases and sentences. Single word gestalts will remain as single word gestalts until a child has gone through the stage 2 mitigation process.

The journey into referential language

Stage 3 consists of isolated single words and word + word combinations. At first there may be a noticeable pause between the words in word + word combinations, as the child is actively processing that these words are linked in meaning. For us to be sure a single word is a stage 3 isolation, we need to see it both in isolation and in combination. For example:

- Octopus.
- Dinosaur.
- Aeroplane.
- Sad.
- Octopus . . . sad.
- Sad . . . octopus.
- Here . . . dinosaur.
- Aeroplane . . . up.

The child may also start to show us that they are obviously noticing individual items, concepts, positions. They may show this by proximity, extended examination of objects or reacting to items as they encounter them. We may see them actively reaching and pointing. We may notice that they are taking time to think before they speak, and when they speak, it is as though they are surprised themselves by the phenomenon of joint-referencing.

We might even observe them contemplating an entity and a word, saying the word to themselves and thinking about it.

For the first time, the child has referential language. Up until now, we couldn't be sure what their concepts were when they used words in phrases. Now they recognise 'car' as a separate entity from the whole experience of being in a car. They have isolated the 'car' from all of its associated sensory experiences or emotional associations. The child's concept of car is similar to ours: 'thing with four wheels; goes on roads; various colours; can be represented by a miniature toy'.

It is possible that older children will explore this stage in their heads. They are aware of how strange this stage appears to other people, and how they sound like a younger child. They may be protecting the adults around them from the panic of thinking that their language has regressed.

What can we offer in this stage?

We can offer a calm presence. We can show that we too can be referential, and we can play with reaching, pointing or showing individual objects, concepts, locations, one at a time. We can play with showing how these individual concepts can also be combined: there are semantic relationships between two words, independent of grammar. This too can be fun.

Each child will enter stage 3 differently, with their particular first isolated word. The word will have been isolated from a stage 2 mitigation, which has been trimmed and trimmed again. For example, if they may have been using stage 2 mitigations 'we can play with the ball', 'we can play with the blocks' and 'we can play with the dog'. Not all of the 'slot' words in this frame will be isolated at the same time; it depends on the child's experiences and language processing. It is possible that from now children do not need to acquire a word via a gestalt to mitigation process, but we need more research in the form of language samples across diverse populations to know more about this.

Intonational variation

Up until now the child's language has been musical with a recognisable intonational pattern for each stage 1 gestalt and stage 2 mitigation. For the first time, a single word has been isolated from the sound curve of the whole phrase. It will sound quite different. It may initially sound quite flat and hesitant, but as a child becomes more secure in stage 3, the intonational pattern of a particular word can start to vary, depending on the intended meaning or language function of the isolated word. So we might hear 'dinosaur' (it's a dinosaur) with a fairly flat intonation, or '*di*nosaur' (I'm so relieved I found it!) with the first syllable stressed, or we might hear 'dinosaur?' (where is my dinosaur? with rising intonation, or 'dinosaur?' (is this really a dinosaur too?) slowed right down with equal stress on each syllable.

Stage 3 also features word + word combinations with associated intonation patterns. For example, the classic 'mummy sock' (this is mummy's sock), '*mummy sock?*' (is this really mummy's sock, and not mine?), 'mummy *sock?*' (is this mummy's sock and not her hat?), '*mummy sock!*' (can you believe it was here?), 'mummy sock?' with rising intonation (where is it?' and 'mummy sock' with falling intonation (it's not here).

When do we start consciously modelling stage 3 language?

If we think that a child is experimenting with stage 3 language, we can join them in pointing at items and entities in our environment and giving them a name. We will gauge the child's response to this. If they find it fun and they join in, we know we are on the right track. If they are naming an item, for example 'cherries', we might copy back their single word and then add an attribute or a location, e.g. 'delicious!'

Richness in stage 2

We also want the child to have enough variety in their stage 1 and stage 2 language.

If we take a language sample and the only stage 2 mitigations we are hearing involve the language chunks 'there's the' and 'it's a', then the child does not yet have the variety for a rich stage 3 experience. Talking naturally with the child for at least 50% of the time, across contexts, with different communication partners, will provide them with that necessary variety.

We don't want to rush the natural process, and so we will wait for them to enter stage 3 naturally, in their own time.

We can model more than one stage

There may well be a period where we are mostly supporting a child in stage 2, but the child also initiates bursts of stage 3 language. Similarly, they may need our support in both stage 3 and stage 4 early experiments with grammar. Stage 3 is very much a crossover stage, which develops concurrently with the stages which precede and follow on. We will need to be flexible in our support, listening carefully to what they say and offering support that matches the stage they are using in this moment.

We don't so much 'model' stage 3 language, as join the child in their stage 3 experiments. We wait for their invitation. When they use a referential word, we join them in this experiment, and we also use a referential word.

Nouns, attributes and locations

When a child has just entered stage 3, we are particularly focused on the following:

- **single noun**, e.g. 'dog', 'chair'

- **single adjective**, e.g. 'wet', 'dirty'

- **noun + noun**, e.g. 'me . . . ball', 'dog . . . chair'

- **adjective + noun**, e.g. 'big . . . dog', 'red . . . ball'

- **noun + adjective**, e.g. 'ball . . . big', 'dog . . . wet'

Then we can start adding some locations into our word + word combinations:

- **location**, e.g. 'there', 'in'

- **noun + location** e.g. 'block . . . here', 'hat . . . off'

- **location + noun** e.g. 'in . . . box', 'there . . . hat'

Once a child is securely within stage 3, i.e. they are regularly using the aforementioned language, we can model the whole range of semantic relationships that can be expressed in two words. We will add in modifiers like 'more', 'no', 'this' and 'those'. For a more comprehensive list, see the section on 'semantic relationships' later in this chapter, and refer to Laura Lee's Developmental Sentence Types (DST)[1] (more on this later).

Stage 3 modelling sounds weird to us, but not to the child

Stage 3 modelling sounds and feels very different, and we need to practice it before we try it with a child. It not only sounds very different from our stage 1 and 2 GLP modelling, but it is also different from the ALP language modelling that we have been trained to do.

Word order does not matter in stage 3

We may have been trained in child-led approaches such as Hanen, Parent-Child Interaction Therapy, VERVE Therapy and Non-Directive Therapy. In all of these approaches we would likely model the correct word order in our two-word combinations. For example, we would model 'big ball' rather than 'ball big'. If I wanted to say the second phrase, we would say 'the ball is big'. We would use grammatical morphemes. We would model 'mummy's here', not 'mummy here'. This is telegraphic language: it does not contain any grammatical morphemes and has completely free word order.

This takes a lot of getting used to. We have to give ourselves permission to model 'incorrect' grammar, and unlearn our previous SLT conditioning.

One way that we are going to accept the sound of ourselves modelling stage 3 language like 'ball big', 'here ball', 'boy ball', is by practising it. We need to get used to how it sounds so that we are not embarrassed. We will need to practise it out loud to ourselves or in front of our pets first, so that we can build up to being comfortable with other people hearing us sound like this: the child we are working with, their parents, teaching staff, other children.

Semantic relationships with no grammar

In stage 3, we are modelling single words, but we are also modelling all the different semantic relationships that can possibly be expressed using only two words. 'Semantics' is word meanings. 'Semantic relationships' is how one word relates in meaning to another word.

We will start just with noun + noun combinations. So look around you, in the room and outside if you are near a window. Think about the relationships between two items, and model stage 3 language using noun + noun combinations.

For me this is:

- table . . . laptop
- me . . . laptop
- dog . . . chair
- chair . . . dog (deliberately practice the word order that sounds odd to you)
- sun . . . sky
- sky . . . sun
- sun . . . plant

Now let's add some adjectives. For me, this feels easier.

- chair . . . soft
- hard . . . table
- warm . . . chair
- dog . . . soft

And then mix it up. Think of all the word + word combinations to express the thoughts you are having about your environment, and the relationship between the entities in your environment.

- laptop . . . table
- chair . . . dog
- warm . . . dog
- sun . . . table
- sun . . . warm

The first few times we do this, there may be some cognitive dissonance. We may say to ourselves that this is easy, whilst simultaneously thinking it is a bit silly and unnecessary. We may revert to only using correct word order when we are with a child. It just feels more right.

The reason that we don't only model 'correct' word order is that we need the child to completely free up each isolated word. We want the child to have the freedom to move each and every word around so that each and every word has come completely 'unstuck' from stage 1 and 2 language. There will be a time for learning grammatical rules, but that is not now. This stage is about word meanings, not grammar.

So we need to stick with it, and keep practising on our own, or perhaps with a pet. We need to get comfortable with this so that we can model stage 3 confidently in front of children and adults in our therapy.

Where are all the verbs?

We wait to model verbs. There are many semantic relationships that we can model before verbs. Verbs are complicated. They have complicated morphology and complicated word order. Verbs are very much linked with grammar. We want to devote our time to word meanings, rather than grammar and word order in stage 3. A stage 3 GLP who has just started isolating words and has just become referential does not need that complexity and pressure at the moment. We want to make their lives easier by focusing on concrete referencing in the here and now.

A variety of semantic relationships

Once a child is securely in stage 3 (we will be able to see this from our language samples) there will be a good variety of single nouns, attributes and locations, and

Table 7.2 Developmental types of pre-sentences (reduced version)

Developmental types of pre-sentences	Examples
Nouns and noun elaborations	Ball, a ball, balls, more balls, this ball, my ball, now ball, daddy ball, big ball, baby ball, ball truck, not ball, another ball? what ball? and ball
Designators and designative elaborations	here, there, this, that, it, those, these, this? here? here ball, these balls, there now, not there, that ball? who that? and here
Other vocabulary items and phrase fragments	Ok, hey, hi, bye-bye, uh-oh, what? In car, for me, plurals, adverbs (all gone, too big, up here), sentence modifications (to you, in it, not big, in here?), conjunctions (and, but)

word + word combinations consisting of these word types. Then we can open the door to more word + word combinations.

Laura Lee's Developmental Sentence Types[2] (DST) is not a familiar tool in the UK but can be used in stages 3 and 4 to chart the different types of semantic relationships in pre-sentences. The complete version is included in the handouts section, but I am providing a much reduced version in Table 7.2, which captures stage 3 pre-sentences and the range of semantic relationships that they explore.

(We will also encounter Lee's Developmental Sentence Analysis[3] in stages 4–6, but in stage 3 we are concerned with pre-sentences.)

Activities for stage 3 modelling

We can use all of the same sensory and movement activities that we have been using in stage 1 and stage 2. These might lend themselves to language like 'light . . . on', 'light . . . off', 'loud . . . quiet', 'fast . . . slow', 'up . . . down' and so on.

Messy play with sand, water, play-dough or gloop offers lots of potential with combinations like 'sand . . . in', 'play-dough . . . soft'.

We can use our construction toys, using single words like 'brick', 'square', 'big', 'little', 'on', 'off', 'red', 'green' and phrases like 'more . . . brick', 'blue . . . circle' and 'no . . . window'.

We can use our pretend-play toys and try out 'this . . . cup', 'that . . . plate', 'cake . . . plate', 'cake . . . on'. We can use the child's favourite characters for exciting adventures and model 'Peppa . . . up', 'up . . . Peppa!' 'George . . . gone', 'there . . . George'. We could feed pretend food to animals and model 'carrot . . . horse', 'cow . . . banana'. We could hide toys in containers and model 'ball . . . box', 'box . . . ball'.

Because stage 3 is referential, we could get out our matching games. For example, Orchard Toys 'Farmyard Heads and Tails' and 'Jungle Jumble'. We can model 'horse . . . horse' when we find a match, and 'lion . . . elephant' when we don't.

We can use our 'Lift-the-Flap' books and interactive books. Nick Sharratt's *Ketchup on Your Cornflakes* is perfect: we can vary intonation to express our likes or dislikes, and how we feel about each combination, e.g. 'custard . . . head?' 'custard . . . bath?' Eric Carle's *The Very Hungry Caterpillar* and *Brown Bear Brown Bear* offer combinations like 'caterpillar . . . ice-cream', 'big . . . caterpillar', 'horse . . . blue', 'yellow . . . duck'. Nick Sharratt and Pippa Goodhart's 'You Choose' series are perfect for stage 3 modelling, especially for older GLPs. Really, we could use any book, magazine or catalogue, taking the child's interests and enthusiasms as our lead.

If the child likes being outside, then we can go on a bug hunt and model 'worm . . . dirty', 'ladybird . . . grass'. We can climb on equipment: 'slide . . . down', 'slide . . . high!'

Short bursts

Stage 3 is hard work. The child is learning a new way of creating novel utterances. We might support stage 3 language in bursts of 5–10 minutes each day, in a variety of situations, to allow a child to explore this stage 3 language. This gives them exposure to a range of referential vocabulary, and a range of semantic relationships.

As always, we need to partner with parents. We will need to agree how we will support a child through this stage. It is entirely possible to apply the NLA protocol through parent coaching. Parents may need a little more support and reassurance through this stage, as the modelling feels less natural. We may need to help explore a wide range of semantic relationships to prepare the child's path into stage 4.

Experimenting with musical aspects

Up until stage 3, the child's language has likely been richly intonational and musical. At the referential stage 3, it can sound a little flat. We may want to experiment with musical qualities in our two-word combinations to see if this appeals to a child. We know from Corinne Zmoos's work[4] that GLPs are often drawn to the musical qualities of language. We may already have discovered that the child is drawn to songs or phrases with musical intervals of an octave, a fourth or a fifth. We might also use these intervals in our modelling of two-word combinations. We might also extend the temporal gap between the first and the second word, to help the child hear the two words separately. As always, we will monitor a child's reaction to this. If it appeals to them, we will keep doing it. If not, we stop.

Don't be tempted to miss out or fly through stage 3!

It may seem as though some children start to use stages 3 and 4 at the same time, or at least in very quick succession. GLPs need time to become secure in this new referential domain. They don't need the pressures of grammar and word order.

If we move on to modelling stage 4 too quickly, a child may conclude that we don't like their hesitant stage 3 and 4 language, and they may revert to their fluent stage 2 language. We need to join them in their stage 3 to show that it is important and it is valued.

The hazy division between late stage 3 and early stage 4

In the case study at the end of this chapter, you will see some examples of late stage 3 and early stage 4 language. We see such a range of pre-sentences towards the end of stage 3 that they start to look like early sentences. Strictly speaking, a sentence has a verb in it. 'There aeroplane' could be a stage 3 pre-sentence, or it could be argued that the intended meaning is 'there is an aeroplane', which is a sentence. I am not convinced that it matters too much: we know that the child is hovering around the end of stage 3 and the beginning of stage 4.

We can refer to Table 4.1 of Chapter 4 to help guide our language modelling. We will continue to just talk naturally for most of the time. With stage 3, we are likely to be modelling a mixture of stages: when the child is using stage 2 language we may add potential mitigations; when they are using stage 3 language we will join them in this; when they use stage 4 language we will listen and acknowledge their early experiments in grammar, without expansion or correction.

Every child's pathway through these stages is marked by unique experiments because their brains are unique and their language processing is unique. Our role is to facilitate their experimentation by keeping the conversation flowing, and communicating that all their language is valued. The scoring of a language sample is ultimately less important than our connection with a child through this process.

If we are listening and acknowledging, perhaps repeating back to corroborate their experiments, we are doing the best we can to partner them through this process.

Summary of stage 3 supports

Stage 3 supports are accompanied by our familiar foundational principles. Supports specific to stage 3 are likely to be in bursts, led by the child. For the rest of the time we are keeping things natural!

- Prioritise trust and connection.

- Keep communication going by doing 'just enough' to keep the connection going.

- Notice when the child is using stage 3 referential language, and otherwise support their language from earlier and later NLA stages.

- Monitor our own regulation. Be unphased when we hear new stage 3 referential language.

- Continue to show our authentic selves. We are still learning, and we can acknowledge this.

- Value and validate all of the child's communication, including gestalts, mitigations and experiments with single words and word + word combinations.

- Partner with parents to ensure that we are all aware of the child's experiments with referential language.

- Talk naturally at least 50% of the time.

- Offer bursts of playful referential language when a child has entered stage 3. We offer noun + noun, noun + attribute and attribute + combinations with free word order.

- Use language that is appealing to the child, perhaps making use of musical intervals in our stage 3 modelling.

- Take regular language samples to track a child's language acquisition, ensuring that the child has fully explored stage 2 mitigations, and have enough language variety to support stage 3 experiments.

- Return to stage 3 for short bursts even when a child is using stage 4 and 5 grammar. Variety in stage 3 is an important foundation for stages 4 and 5.

How we track progress in stage 3

We will look at the variety of semantic relationships being expressed. We can use the DST, or the reduced version in this chapter, to highlight any gaps. We can then think about which activities we might offer that will provide natural opportunities to model particular semantic relationships. For example, if a child is using a lot of colour words but no other attributes, we might get out toys that demonstrate an obvious size difference, to offer opportunities to model 'cake . . . big' and 'little . . . cup'. If a child is not using many location words, we might play a hiding and finding game, which will allow us to model 'ball . . . here' and 'there . . . ball'.

Goals for a stage 3 GLP

A child may stop off in stage 3 for a very short time, and so we may write a stage 3 goal alongside a stage 2 or a stage 4 goal.

The support that a child needs in stage 3 will vary enormously: younger children and dual processors are likely to whizz through this stage quickly, but older students may need to spend longer there.

A stage 3 goals might be written as:

> *When involved in a well-regulating, quiet situation, with a playful and GLP- informed communication partner, Jack will spontaneously produce single words and/or unique word + word combinations 50% of the time.*

> *When given unrestricted access to regulatory supports, and with a supportive communication partner, Jack will use stage 3 single words and word + word combinations as part of a rich mix of NLA language stages.*

Case study: Jack

Jack first came to see me in my clinic a month before he turned 4. He literally bounced into the room, with his red hair and denim dungarees, and enthusiastically engaged with all the toys I had got out.

Jack loved phrases with a dramatic intonation, and frequently swooped on toys saying, 'look at this!' with an excited gasp. If he heard an environmental sound he would ask, 'what's that noise?' with wide eyes. Other gestalts included 'I got it!' 'jump jump jump', 'mummy do it?' counting up to 5 and down from 5, 'ready steady go!' and several songs, including 'Zoom zoom zoom' and 'Five little monkeys'.

I heard a few single words in our first session, including 'cat', 'orange', 'red', 'triangle', 'square', 'circle', 'oval' and 'rectangle'. I did not hear these single words in any other combination, be it a gestalt, a mitigation, a two-word combination or an early sentence, and so for now I scored these as stage 1 gestalts, even though they appeared to be referential.

Language samples taken over the next two weeks suggested that Jack was largely in stage 1, and that he would benefit from more variety in his stage 1 language, in terms of form and content, and communication intentions. He had a lot of gestalts for engaging the attention of his communication partner, some lovely reciprocal games and songs, and one gestalt, 'mummy do it?' for requesting help. I advised his family to just keep the conversation going, occasionally adding new ideas, but largely following Jack's train of thought, and speaking what they thought he would like to say.

In our sessions together, I experimented with offering language around describing, e.g. 'it's enormous!'; expressing joy, 'I love it!'; expressing sensory needs, 'let's hop'; talking about transitions, 'it's nearly time to finish'; requesting help, 'need some help'; and protesting, 'I don't like it'. Since Jack loved the dramatic, I tried to use as animated a voice as I could, with big pitch intervals and comedy voices. Jack responded to these with a smile and often eye contact. He used the language I offered very readily, with us taking equal turns in interactions.

Stage 2 mitigations began to emerge. Jack's gestalt 'mummy do it?' began to be mixed with 'Jack do it!' His gestalt 'it's a dinosaur!' was freely combined with a huge range of nouns like 'it's a helicopter!' 'it's a octopus!' and 'it's a mummy!' I noticed that Jack's stage 2 language often took the form of 'frames-and-slots'. From the start, his stage 1 language had been fairly transparent: there weren't a lot of media gestalts, but rather the language that he had heard from his family whilst playing. He did love songs, and I noticed that these were being mitigated by swopping words in and out, e.g. 'I see triceratops' and 'I see stegosaurus', as well as whole songs being trimmed down line by line.

Jack entered school. Our sessions moved to school, with different teaching staff joining us each session, so that they could get a feel for how to support him in class. Staff noticed how playful and communicative Jack was in these sessions. Hearing his rich varied language helped them to view him as a very intentional communicator who was making connections between different experiences. I would hear Jack chatting with them as he came up the corridor: he clearly had a good connection with his teaching assistants.

Jack's stage 2 mitigations became more varied, with phrases like 'where are you [noun]?', 'there's a [noun]', 'get the [noun]', 'is it a [noun]?', 'it's [adjective]', 'that's . . . [adjective]', 'it's . . . [adjective], 'let's . . . [verb], and 'we can [verb]'.

By my eighth session with Jack, I was confident from my language samples that Jack's single words were stage 3 isolations. Jack used words including 'purple', 'red', 'yellow', 'dinosaur', 'helicopter', 'aeroplane', 'rocket', 'duck' and 'cat' both in isolation and in combination.

Jack loved playing with little sorting dinosaurs, pretend food and some little presents that each contained a miniature toy. I tried out some short bursts of referential naming and labelling attributes. For example, 'dinosaur . . . red', 'strawberry . . . cake', 'cake . . . plate', 'aeroplane . . . little', 'aeroplane . . . box', 'up . . . aeroplane!' Jack joined in with this for a few turns, and then returned to his stage 1 and 2 language. In class, Jack's teaching assistants continued to talk naturally for most of the time, but modelling stage 2 mitigations when the opportunity arose.

Over the next couple of weeks I varied our toys so that we had rich and varied language material to work with. Jack always gravitated towards his favourites (dinosaurs, pretend food and presents) but also explored other toys in short bursts. I brought in animals, vehicles and sensory toys that were 'soft', 'squishy', 'spiky', 'shiny', 'wet', 'sticky', 'loud', 'fast' and 'scary'. We looked at the 'You Choose' book and Jack picked out 'rocket', 'hot air balloon', 'parachute'. Jack especially liked a reversible octopus and would say 'octopus happy!' and 'octopus sad' as he changed it.

Jack had already started to use a few isolated verbs, including 'help', 'fly', 'go' and 'stop'. Whilst I repeated these utterances, I didn't model them in word + word combinations yet.

Almost at the same time, Jack started to use some stage 4 language mixed in with his stage 3. For example, 'it a helicopter' (stage 4) alongside 'a helicopter', *'it helicopter' (late stage 3). I could track Jack's isolation of words within the same language sample, where I might hear 'where's the dinosaur?' (stage 2 mitigation); 'dinosaur', 'dinosaur there' (stage 3); 'where the dinosaur?', 'a dinosaur there', 'there a dinosaur', 'there the dinosaur' (stage 4).*

Language samples were a fascinating record of language development. I have re-ordered these utterances from a single session to show the mix of stages, and the journey of specific words from a modelled gestalt through to stage 4 language:

> *'The aeroplane's flying!' – 0 [copied from my modelling]*
>
> *'The aeroplane's flying!' – 1 [used spontaneously later in the session]*
>
> *'aeroplane's flying!' – 2 [trimmed down mitigation]*
>
> *'flying!' – 2 [trimmed further]*
>
> *'aeroplane' – 2 [tentative scoring, later changed to 3 when seen in combination]*
>
> *'aeroplane duck' – 3 [the aeroplane picked up the duck in a rescue mission!]*
>
> *'there aeroplane' – 3*
>
> *'here aeroplane' – 3*
>
> *'no aeroplane' – 3*
>
> *'this is aeroplane' – 4*

Jack's language showed an explosion at this point. His family noted that he was saying new words and phrases every day, in new combinations that had not been modelled. For example, they drove past school on a weekend and Jack said, 'Hello school! Hello friends!'

Jack still used a lot of stage 1 and 2 language. He was still acquiring new language gestalts, and then trimming them down. We would hear a stream of stage 1 gestalts together in a moment of high excitement. Jack had always enjoyed sound effects in his play, and it was not unusual to have a significant portion of a language sample made up of noises like 'RAH!' from Tyrannosaurus Rex and hurt sounds or scared sounds of other dinosaurs. His stage 1 gestalts were important in his play, for 'run away!' and 'oh no, hide here!' and 'VOLCANO!' Stage 1 language like 'ok, I'll help you' (used as a request for help) also seemed to be easier for Jack to access in a hurry.

I had to be very careful to slow myself down when playing with Jack. I knew that my therapy heritage of non-directive therapy meant that I was sometimes over-eager to model new language. In stages 3 and 4, Jack needed time to formulate what he was going to say. He often hesitated in mid-air: all of his movements would stop, and I could see him actively processing. I got to know that some stage 3 or 4 language was brewing by this characteristic pause.

I used Laura Lee's DST to check that I was modelling a wide range of semantic relationships. I realised we needed to spend some time with locations, e.g. 'up aeroplane', 'helicopter in'. Then other modifiers: 'more dinosaur', 'this triceratops', 'where stegosaurus?' 'stegosaurus there'. Interestingly, Jack did not copy this back in the same session, but often in subsequent sessions he seemed to have integrated it, and used the same words in stage 4 language, for example 'stegosaurus in there' and 'where the red gone?'

Twelve months after I had met him, Jack now had a good foundation for early experiments with grammar in stage 4.

Notes

1 Lee, L. (1966) 'Developmental sentence types: A method for comparing normal and deviant syntactic development' *Journal of Speech and Hearing Disorders*. With thanks to Northwestern University Press for their permission to reproduce the DST and DSS in this book.

2 Lee, L. (1966) 'Developmental sentence types: A method for comparing normal and deviant syntactic development' *Journal of Speech and Hearing Disorders*. With thanks to Northwestern University Press for their permission to reproduce the DST and DSS in this book.

3 Lee, L. (1974) *Developmental Sentence Analysis: A Grammatical Assessment Procedure for Speech and Language Clinicians* Northwestern University Press.

4 https://www.crescendocommunication.com/

Chapter 8

Stage 4
Generation of first sentences

Revision: the six stages of Natural Language Acquisition

We have come a long way! We have seen the child make the leap into referential language. Stage 3 was all about semantics. Now we get into grammar, in the context of meaningful interactions. We are in sentence territory. This is a brave step for a child. They are intentionally converting the thoughts that are in their head into grammatical constructions that we will understand.

Table 8.1 The six stages of Natural Language Acquisition

		Examples
Stage 1	Language gestalts (wholes, scripts, songs, language soundtracks from experiences)	Zoom zoom zoom, we're going to the moon! It's a dinosaur!
Stage 2	Mitigations: a) Shortening long gestalts b) Dividing them into chunks c) Recombining different chunks	We're going to the moon! We're going! We're going to the shops! It's an octopus!
Stage 3	Isolated single words Word + word combinations of referential single words	dinosaur; rocket dinosaur . . . big; rocket . . . up
Stage 4	Original phrases and beginning sentences	We got dinosaur Put rocket up there
Stage 5	Original sentences with more complex grammar	I can get the dinosaurs I don't want to put my shoes on
Stage 6	Original sentences culminating in a complete grammar system	Who could have taken the dinosaurs? I've been looking for my shoes

DOI: 10.4324/9781032717029-8

How do we know when a child is moving into stage 4?

We can be confident that a child has reached stage 4 if we have been carefully tracking their language samples and we have seen a clear move through earlier stages. Our language samples will ideally have shown an earlier period where stage 2 made up at least 50% of their utterances, and a clear stage 3 referencing period. We were able to see variety in these stages: they could express a wide range of communication intentions in stage 2, and they explored a wide range of semantic relationships in stage 3 (see p. 96).

How do we distinguish between highly flexible stage 2 language and stage 4 language?

If we haven't partnered a child through their stage 2 and stage 3 language, this can be tricky. It is easy to confuse stage 2 with stage 4.

Clues that an utterance is stage 2 are its fluency and musicality: it will have retained part of the intonational curve from the stage 1 gestalt. Stage 4 language is likely to, at least initially, sound more effortful or hesitant. It will not flow as fluently as all the stage 2 language we have been accustomed to hearing.

However, a child may be well within their stage 4 journey, and so may sound reasonably fluent. How do we know then?

The best way of determining if the language we are hearing is stage 4 or language from an earlier stage is to take a language sample, or a couple of language samples. Wait until a child is comfortable partnering with us, before we take this language sample. Collaborate with the parent so that they can help us score the language sample. They will likely recognise stage 1 and stage 2 language and can correct our scoring if we have scored these utterances as stage 4.

Examine the language sample carefully. Have the words that appear in the language sample been successfully freed up? Are they being used flexibly as single units within a few different utterances? If they have, it is likely that we are seeing stage 4 language.

There may well be a few 'mini-chunks': word combinations that always seem to appear together. This is not to say that the child is not using stage 4 language, just that there are still a few residual mini-chunks in and amongst words that have been completely freed.

Take the extract from a language sample in Table 8.2, from Sam.

Focus on the word 'put'. This appears initially to only appear in a 'mini-chunk' as 'put in'. However later in the language sample (utterance 45 and beyond) it appears

Table 8.2 Stage 4 language sample showing isolated flexible words

35	S	Don't put it in oven!		4
	A	Oh, don't put it in the oven?		
36	S	Don't put mine . . . put my oven glove		4
	A	Oh, good idea. Put it on.		
37	S	What do we need?	Sam was looking for the other oven glove	1
	A	Oh, we need another one!		
	M	I think you can do it with one hand, can't you sweet?	Sam conceded that he could manage with one oven glove!	
38	S	Have to put in oven		4
	A	Have to put in oven		
39	S	Put in oven		4
	A	Put in oven		
40	S	Put in the oven		4
	A	Put in the oven. The oven is hot.		
(The language sample has been reduced for the purpose of demonstration.)				
45	S	Put on		4
	A	Put on . . . the plate		
46	S	Put candles		4
	A	Oh yes, don't forget them!		
47	S	Put the candles		4
	A	Yes. Put the candles . . . on the cake		

in other combinations too: 'put on', 'put candles' and 'put the candles'. We can also see in the language sample that many other words are being used flexibly as single units in a phrase or sentence.

This extract is from a full language sample which shows many other utterances where isolated words are being used flexibly in a variety of constructions. We will always look at a whole language sample (or multiple language samples) to check that this is part of a bigger picture of stage 4 language use.

If we are not confident that the child has thoroughly passed through stages 2 and 3, or if the child's language samples are not showing variety in earlier stages, we will want to model more language from that earlier stage for a little longer. Refer to the 'Language supports at different stages of NLA' refer to Table 4.1 in Chapter 4 if we are unsure from a language sample which stage we should be focusing on.

Stage 4 is where grammar begins

Stage 3 language was free of grammar. It was about the semantic relationships between two referential words. Stage 4 is the child's first experiments with grammar: with word order, with grammatical elements like pronouns, verb forms, negatives and questions, and with grammatical morphemes like the -s ending of plurals and the correct verb ending.

Stage 4 begins by sounding simple, but by the end of stage 4 a child is able to produce a wide range of sentence types. They can signal whether they are talking about something in the past, present or future. They can specify who was involved. They can ask a variety of questions, and they can begin to clarify aspects of their message in the event of a misunderstanding.

Examples of early stage 4 language include:

- Me go now.
- No like it.
- Where it is?
- Car in there.
- You me do it.
- It big one.

There may be grammatical morphemes, as the child starts to learn the rules of grammar. We will see the sorts of grammatical errors or overgeneralisations that we are used to seeing in ALP children. For example:

- It comed out!

- These sheeps are eating.

We will probably see some 'mini-chunks' left over from stage 2. These are chunks of language that have not yet been completely broken down. The mini-chunks are shown in brackets as follows:

- (I'm gonna) take this one.

- (It's) a (really big) pile here.

- Mummy, do you want a (really big) one?

When we notice that these are mini-chunks, we circle them on our language sample, so that we know that at some point we need to come back to them and model in isolation. For example, in order to break up the mini-chunk of it's, we might later model 'it's over there . . . is it? *It is!*'

Mazing

Because the child is actively processing grammar, we will likely see them pause and struggle over their grammatical constructions and word order. We may see a phenomenon known as 'mazing'. This is linguistic dysfluency, rather than speech dysfluency, but they can sound very similar. We may hear the child repeat fragments or chunks of language. They may actively re-order words or change morphemes mid-utterance. It can sound a little like stammering, but this is a linguistic phenomenon rather than a speech motor phenomenon. Some examples include:

- (I'm gonna) (I'm gonna) I'm gonna to put that here.

- (He's not) (he's not) she's not dancing now.

- They're . . . (ok, ok) (they're m . . .) making peanut butter sandwiches.

The child needs time to think through exactly which word they need next, possibly including a relatively new grammatical morpheme. They may need to change or re-order the words mid-utterance. They may be aware that they need to modify their phrase or sentence so that it better reflects their communication intention.

This is hard work! We need to respect the child's processing time. We can slow our own pace, stay present, and manage our own regulation at these times. We might need to reassure parents that this is normal in stage 4. It reflects the huge shift into grammar, as the child adopts analytic strategies into their language processing in order to produce novel utterances from isolated words.

Moving from pre-sentences into early sentences

You might remember Laura Lee's 'Developmental Sentence Types' (DST) from stage 3 (see p. 97). The DST continues to be useful in stage 4, as the child starts producing more elaborate pre-sentences. Stage 3 pre-sentences were two-word combinations. Now we might see these pre-sentences (Table 8.3, adapted from Lee[1] and Blanc[2]):

Table 8.3 Developmental types of pre-sentences (reduced)

Developmental types of pre-sentences	Examples
Nouns and noun elaborations	my big car, all of them, some other cars, now the car, the car the garage, all of mine, not that one, the other car? which other one? how many cars? and the car; car and truck
Designative elaborations	here another car, there another car, this a red car, it my truck, here some cars, here car now, there mummy daddy, that somebody car, here his car, that not car, that a car? who that boy? what that one?
Descriptive elaborations	the car broken, the light on, car in garage, all cars broken, light off now, truck too dirty, it clean now, this not broken, it off now? where that one? who in car? what colour car? car and truck here?
Verb elaborations	eat the biscuit, put the table, take off hat, turn on light, the car go, a boy eat, goes in house, want it now, not fall down, see that one? eat more biscuit? where put car? what take out? what find here? what doing to car? and find car

The full version of Laura Lee's DST can also be found in the handouts section.

We also see first sentences in stage 4. Marge Blanc's Natural Language Acquisition Protocol recommends that we use another framework from Laura Lee, Developmental Sentence Scoring (DSS).[3] The DSS spans the earliest stage 4 sentence constructions, through to stage 6 constructions. The DSS is organised into eight levels. Lee's levels 1 to 3 equate to NLA stage 4. Lee's levels 4 to 6 equate to NLA stage 5, and levels 7 and 8 are NLA stage 6 (Table 8.4).

Quick reference comparing DSS levels with NLA stages

Table 8.4 Quick reference comparing DSS levels with NLA stages

DSS levels	NLA stage
1–3	4
4–6	5
7–8	6

I'm just going to issue a health warning here. The DSS will look completely overwhelming at first. But remember, Laura Lee captured pretty much all the sentence types that are possible across complete language acquisition.

Stage 4 is just concerned with DSS levels 1–3.

We do not need to memorise the DSS, but it will be invaluable to have a copy handy, as we will refer to it in our language samples from now on. The DSS is included in the handouts section of this book, and it can be downloaded for free from the Communication Development Center website.

Just like with any other tool we use in Speech and Language Therapy, we will become familiar with the DSS when we use it with specific children we work with.

Our language samples will show that a child's stage 4 language is naturally showing some of the constructions in levels 1–3 of the DSS. They tend to appear in the sequence that Laura Lee describes. If we see one particular construction from level 1, we will likely see more pop up naturally. We can model other constructions at this level.

We might also see constructions from levels 2 and 3. Just like the stages of NLA, a child does not neatly move linearly from one level to the next. There will be a mixture. But the levels do roughly follow a progression.

The pronouns 'you' and 'I' may come later

The DSS is a tool based on ALP grammar development. It may be that there are differences in GLP grammar development: we will only know this over time with more research. The pronouns 'you' and 'I' may take longer to resolve. This is not, as we might have said previously, because this language is 'disordered'. It is just because a GLP may have acquired gestalts with these pronouns and now they have to work out that the pronouns were reversed. This may take time.

Similarly other pronouns may slightly lag behind other grammatical constructions as the child moves through the DSS. Anecdotally, in my practice, I find that the pronouns 'he' and 'she' (and 'his', 'her' and 'hers') take a little longer to appear. A child may be well into stage 5 before these appear. I would not particularly worry about this; maybe little GLPs are leading the way in showing us that gendered pronouns are not particularly needed!

Have the DST or DSS available on the fridge!

It is helpful to have the DST or DSS visible. Once a child has explored a wide variety of semantic relationships from the DST, we begin to use the DSS. We might print out a copy for the family to stick on their fridge and the teaching staff to have on the classroom wall. If the whole DST or DSS seems overwhelming, then we might cut this down to the parts we are particularly interested in at this time.

Having the DST or DSS on display makes it more likely that adults will notice or use these constructions in natural interactions with the child. When we hear a particular construction, we might scribble it down, or ask the parent or teacher to scribble it down. Having the DSS visible also reminds us of all the work the child is doing internally, and why they need that extra processing time.

Keep on partnering with the child

Our most important task is, as ever, to keep the connection going. The child is leading the way, with their play and with their language. We are here to listen, to acknowledge their language in a way that we know they like and to help them express the ideas that are in their head. As they move through stage 4, children may struggle to put into words the complex and nuanced ideas that are in their heads. There may be misunderstandings. By repeating back what we heard, we can help a child to identify whether we need more information. We are giving them extra processing time by not adding any new language for now.

There are some grammatical developments that help a child clear up misunderstandings now. They start to use negatives and question forms. So for the first time we can be confident that they will correct us, e.g. 'not jumping, *running*'. We can check back with them by using rising intonation to question what they want or mean, e.g. 'this one?' or 'the pizza slice?' We can also reinforce their ideas quite naturally, e.g. 'oh yes, it *is*', all very naturally modelling stage 4 constructions.

We may need to be more thorough for older GLPs

For a younger child who has been moving through the NLA stages quite quickly and easily, we can take a fairly relaxed approach to supporting stage 4 language. We continue with all children to just talk naturally for at least 50% of the time.

We can check in with the DSS, give the relevant handout to those who are going to be modelling language and assume that this will provide the variety that the child needs. We can check this every now and again with our language samples.

For an older child who might have been late to Natural Language Acquisition, we might want to be more thorough and make sure that we are modelling each structure in the DSS.

To make this call, we will be considering how dynamic the child's language growth is. If they are creating new language every day we will need a less prescriptive approach, similar to a young child. If their language samples show that they have a restricted variety of stage 4 language, we might focus our modelling on particular constructions and monitor their uptake. But we don't ever want it to sound like we are drilling or eliciting language.

Avoiding the child's stage 2 language?

For children who have spent a long time in stage 2, we may choose to avoid their favourite phrase starters when we are consciously supporting stage 4 language. For example, if a child loves to mitigate phrases with 'it's' or 'we're' or 'let's' at the start of their phrases, we might try not to use these constructions. Stage 2 language will be very comfortable for them now, compared with the word + word + word effortful stage 4 language they are grappling with. If we are using a lot of their favourite stage 2 language, we are not helping them make this leap into self-generated 'building up from scratch' grammar.

We don't correct child's early experiments with grammar

The child's language has undergone a huge shift in stage 3. They have become referential. Now they are for the first time actively building a phrase or sentence, word by word. This takes tremendous processing effort. We want to acknowledge this effort by listening. We don't then correct their mistakes! They will have time to iron out their grammatical errors. The DST and DSS show us the vast array of pre-sentence types and sentence constructions that a child is exploring in this stage. When we appreciate the scale of the work the child is undertaking we realise that the child already has more than enough to do, without us adding suggestions for improvement. We are here to partner in this process, not to lead the child or direct the child.

But we can help them out if we see that they are struggling

There will be times when the child is struggling to convey the ideas they have in their head into grammatical language. If we see that they are struggling, and if it feels natural for us to supply the phrase or sentence that they are searching for, we might cautiously offer this to them. We will gauge their reaction to this. We don't want to do this too often, and we certainly don't want to jump in too early when they were actively building a sentence. As with previous stages, videoing our sessions will be invaluable. We can watch back what happened, and judge whether we are using the right supports at this time.

We can add to what they say

We can also judiciously use the strategy of adding on to their utterance. We didn't 'copy and add' to their utterances in the earlier stages because we understood that until a child has isolated words themselves, they will not be able to just add another word to their stage 1 or stage 2 language. Now we can support them by just doing what feels natural, so that if a child says, 'people going home now', we might naturally say, 'yes, they're going home on the bus'. Again, we will monitor a child's response to this: if they don't like what we're doing, we rethink it.

Summary of stage 4 supports

- Continue to prioritise trust and connection.

- Keep communication going by doing 'just enough'.

- Allow silence and space for the child to think and process language.

- Monitor our own regulation. Keep calm and give time when the child is 'mazing'.

- Continue to show our authentic selves. We are having conversations; we bring our real experiences to these.

- Value and validate all of the child's communication, including gestalts, mitigations, their experiments with single words and two-word combinations, and their early experimental grammar. We don't try to correct or improve this in any way.

- Partner with parents to ensure that we are all aware of the child's experiments with grammar, and what the child may be trying to convey with their early grammar experiments.

- Talk naturally at least 50% of the time.

- Take regular language samples to track a child's language acquisition, using the DST and DSS to identify constructions that a child is naturally exploring.

- Note any 'mini-chunks' that are left over from stage 2, and modelling these words separately from one another.

- Provide models of particular grammatical constructions only where a child seems to need these, if they have spent some time in stage 4.

- Use the DST and then the DSS to guide us in particular language that the child has yet to acquire.

How we track progress in stage 4

We will continue to take regular language samples to track a child's journey through stage 4, from the emergence of the first original phrases and beginning sentences, through to increasing variety in grammatical constructions. We will look for the variety of stage 4 language, looking at the different elements of the DSS, e.g. indefinite and personal pronouns, verb constructions, negatives, questions. When report writing, we might compile a table like Table 8.5 to consider the variety in grammatical constructions:

Table 8.5 Tracking variety in grammatical constructions

Stage 4 grammar	Examples from language samples	Next steps
Indefinite pronouns: it, that, this	Get **it, that,** look at **this**	Stage 5 indefinite pronouns: nothing, nobody, none

(Continued)

Stage 4 grammar	Examples from language samples	Next steps
Personal pronouns: I, you, me, my, your	**I** want play, **me** make pizza, **we** get laptop	Personal pronouns: 'you', 'my'
Main verbs: eat, eating	**Jump**, **make** a cake, **open** it up, **take** a piece, **eat** pizza, **look** at those strawberries, we **get** laptop	Further variety in main verbs and in verb tenses, e.g. past tense, present progressive (verb+ing)
Secondary verbs: want **to get** it, going **to eat** it	I want **play**, need **cut**	Further variety in secondary verbs
Negatives, e.g. not	**No** tissue, laptop **gone**, **can't** reach it	Use of 'not', e.g. 'not red'
Conjunctions, e g. and	Not yet observed in stage 4 language	Use of 'and', e.g. 'mushrooms and peppers'
Reversals, e.g. is it? Are you?	Not yet observed in stage 4 language	Use of reversals, e.g. 'is it hot?'
Wh- questions, e.g. 'what is it?'	**Where's** birthday cake?	Further question forms, e.g. what?, who?

Goals for a stage 4 GLP

As already noted, stage 4 is huge, and sounds very different at the start of stage 4 to how it sounds at the end of stage 4. We will again write SCRUFFY goals, allowing for Natural Language Acquisition.

An early stage 4 goal might be written as:

When involved in a well-regulating, quiet situation, with a playful and GLP- informed communication partner, Alex will use a wide variety of pre-sentences, as set out in Laura Lee's Developmental Sentence Types (1966). These will include noun elaborations (my big car, car and truck), descriptive elaborations (a dirty truck, this truck broken) and verb elaborations (me eat this, car gone where?).

A late stage 4 goal might be written as:

When involved in a well-regulating, quiet situation, with a playful and GLP- informed communication partner, Alex will use a variety of early sentence types, as set out in Laura Lee's Developmental Sentence Analysis (1974). This includes using determiners (the, a, this, it), personal pronouns (I, you, he, she), early verb constructions (walking, eating, walked, ate), negatives 'no, not' and the conjunction 'and'.

Case study: Alex

Alex's parents contacted me because his school SLT had identified that he was a GLP. This had been transformational for the family, and they had attended the Meaningful Speech course for parents online.

Alex's parents were also in discussion with Alex's mainstream school about how they could best support him. They were concerned that Alex's EHCP contained references to approaches such as 'Attention Autism', PECS and Colourful Semantics. They were not sure whether these approaches were compatible with NLA, or suitable for Alex as a GLP.

Alex's mum told me before our first meeting that Alex was producing stage 3 and 4 language but at school was mainly using stage 1 and 2 language. His parents had identified that he may not yet have enough stage 1 and 2 language variety. For instance, he did not yet have language for expressing joy or protesting.

Alex's parents sent me some videos of him at home and in the garden using his natural language. His mum also shared a language sample from home.

Alex was also accessing support from a sensory integration trained Occupational Therapist, with a focus upon vestibular and proprioceptive supports.

I had to be very quiet in our first few sessions, to build trust with Alex. I knew that he was finding school difficult due to sensory regulation needs.

Within a couple of sessions, Alex was sharing some of his stage 1 gestalts, many of which were songs like 'Ten in the Bed' and acting out whole sequences from Julia Donaldson stories like 'Room on the Broom'. Alex's gestalts generally involved whole body movements, acting out the dramatic scenes. He loved the actions of falling and dropping items, or rolling them off surfaces. Alex was also mitigating from many of his stage 1 gestalts.

A series of utterances initially confused me: Alex picked up marbles in turn and said 'one purple', 'two blue' and so on, but the colours of the marbles did not correlate to the colour he was saying. Alex used this gestalt in many of our subsequent sessions, but it started to be mitigated with various items, and then the colour started to match the item. It was only much later in our sessions that Alex showed me the original source of this gestalt, in a 'Dino' YouTube clip.

Early on, I did not get 50 utterances in one session, and so my language samples consisted of both what I was hearing in our sessions and language that Alex's parents collected and sent to me. These language samples initially showed that Alex would benefit from more variety in his stage 2 mitigations.

Then Alex started to reveal stage 3 isolations and combinations. Initially these consisted of a colour plus a noun, for example, 'purple gift', 'purple drink', 'green gift', 'green bear'. Over the next few months, Alex's parents and I added bursts of stage 3 modelling into our interactions with him. Alex's dad especially enjoyed this game, and armed with the DST, he did a wonderful job in fully exploring pre-sentences in a variety of situations. Soon I was seeing this in Alex's language samples, with utterances including 'that', 'that one', 'gone', 'broken', 'no tissue', 'chocolate . . . cake', 'yummy . . . delicious', 'watermelon . . . watermelon', 'green . . . red' (comparing two items).

It was clear that Alex was putting a lot of thought into his language: he looked at an item carefully, took some time to think, and then announced his language.

Alex loves drawing, and produces beautiful bright works of art. Interestingly, at this time, his drawings focused on one item at a time: the same items that appeared in his language samples: a watermelon, a pizza, a cake, a rocket and so on.

At the same time, we heard stage 4 emerge, with utterances such as 'not yellow . . . pink!' and 'get chocolate', 'we play', 'make a cake', 'look, laptop, find it', 'open it up . . . squish', 'get pizza' and 'let's put here'.

Sometimes it was tricky to work out whether an utterance was a stage 2 mix-and-match or a stage 4 completely self-generated utterance. Alex was still adding to his stage 1 and stage 2 language, and this was increasingly flexible and varied. Sometimes we could identify that a new utterance was stage 2 because we recognised an intonation pattern. Generally, stage 2 language was more fluent, whereas stage 3 and 4 language was very deliberate, with a flatter intonation, and the words sounding more separate.

Alex's mum sent me an update each week, which included what the family had been doing, the sorts of play Alex was enjoying, what he was singing, watching, drawing, reading and writing, and also what he had said. One of her updates included the following:

Friday – really enjoying 'spinning' in the garden (he copies this from Peter Rabbit 2 but definitely fulfils a sensory need). He rolled over a mound of grass in the garden. Alex fell off the top of a plastic car. Cut his eyebrow and still wearing the plaster. Very sad but did really well at communicating his needs and feelings 'Alex ouchie. Alex sad. Hurt the eye. Need a plaster!' Later in the day he said, 'Alex fell outside' 'Alex fly in the sky. Hurt the face'.

Alex's language samples showed a mix of stages, sometimes showing active breaking down from a gestalt to a mitigation to an isolated word. For example, in this extract from a language sample (Table 8.6):

Table 8.6 Alex's language sample 1

36	Alex	It's strawberries	4
37	Alex	Strawberries to the cake	4
38	Alex	It's strawberries	4
	Ali	It's strawberries	
39	Alex	It strawberries	3

(Continued)

40	Alex	Look at those strawberries	4
41	Alex	Some . . . some . . . it's a candle	4
	Ali	Oh, some candles	
42	Alex	candle	3
43	Alex	Happy Birthday!	2

At this point, Alex was producing many more utterances in a session. We could see an explosion in vocabulary, and in pre-sentence and sentence types.

Alex began to show me where a gestalt had come from. We would often begin our session with the iPad on YouTube Kids, with Alex showing me favourite video clips. He would then act out some of these songs and clips, and I could see him whittling it down to isolate the word he was interested in. For example, in this extract from a language sample (Table 8.7):

Table 8.7 Alex's language sample 2

13	Alex	Five little speckled frogs sat on a speckled log Eating some most delicious bugs – yum yum One jumped into the pool Where it was nice and cool Then there were four green specked frogs	Singing this with 5 squishy balls	1
14	Alex	Three little speckled frogs sat on a speckled log Eating some most delicious bugs – yum yum One jump	Made one of the balls jump onto the trampoline	2
	Ali	Jump in the pool		
16	Alex	jump		4

Alex's mum continued to provide weekly updates, such as:

> *Wednesday speech samples:*
>
> *'where are the glasses? – you get it' (asking me to find my glasses)*
>
> *'Star Wars is gone – need to fix it' (asking to watch Star Wars IV – it's scratched!)*
>
> *'Star Wars number 4 is broken'*
>
> *'The purple one – found it!' (Playing with magnetic tiles)*
>
> *'got it – it's dark' (looking outside)*
>
> *'it broke – help me – oh no!'*
>
> *'Dropped it – mummy get it'*

and a couple of months later:

> *'The black train! It's missing.*
>
> *It must be somewhere.*
>
> *We can't find it.*
>
> *Oh no!*
>
> *Yes! The black train! We found it!'*

As Alex moved through stage 4 the variety of his language naturally increased. His communication felt more 'back-and-forth' and so was naturally more conversational. This allowed the adults around him to add just enough to his ideas to add more variety to his repertoire.

Notes

1 Lee, L. (1966) 'Developmental sentence types: A method for comparing normal and deviant syntactic development' *Journal of Speech and Hearing Disorders*. With thanks to Northwestern University Press for their permission to reproduce the DST and DSS in this book.

2 Blanc, M. (2012) *Natural Language Acquisition on the Autism Spectrum: The Journey from Echolalia to Self-Generated Language*. Communication Development Center, p. 42.

3 Lee, L. (1974) *Developmental Sentence Analysis: A Grammatical Assessment Procedure for Speech and Language Clinicians* Northwestern University Press. With thanks to Northwestern University Press for their permission to reproduce the DST and DSS in this book.

Chapter 9

Stages 5 and 6

Complex grammar to complete grammar

Revision: the stages of Natural Language Acquisition

Stage 4 was a huge stage, spanning pre-sentence grammar through to early sentences. Stages 5 and 6 continue the journey into more sophisticated grammar (Table 9.1). This naturally happens as a child feels the desire to express more complicated or more nuanced meanings.

Table 9.1 The six stages of Natural Language Acquisition

		Examples
Stage 1	Language gestalts (wholes, scripts, songs, language soundtracks from experiences)	Zoom zoom zoom, we're going to the moon! It's a dinosaur!
Stage 2	Mitigations: a) Shortening long gestalts b) Dividing them into chunks c) Recombining different chunks	We're going to the moon! We're going! We're going to the shops! It's an octopus!
Stage 3	Isolated single words Word + word combinations of referential single words	dinosaur; rocket dinosaur . . . big; rocket . . . up
Stage 4	Original phrases and beginning sentences	We got dinosaur Put rocket up there
Stage 5	Original sentences with more complex grammar	I can get the dinosaurs I don't want to put my shoes on
Stage 6	Original sentences culminating in a complete grammar system	Who could have taken the dinosaurs? I've been looking for my shoes

DOI: 10.4324/9781032717029-9

Why do we need to use complex grammar?

Grammar is the tool we use to express increasingly complex or nuanced ideas. Grammar allows us to modulate meaning with ever more subtle shifts of emphasis. For example, compare the following sentences, and the modulations of meaning that are signalled through grammar.

- I want to do it.

- I want to do it myself.

- I will go to the party.

- I may go to the party but I'm not sure yet.

- Although I think I'd like to go to the party, I'm not sure that I have the energy, and if I go and don't like it, how do I get home?

The subtle art of supporting later stages

An attuned communication partner will recognise when a child is trying to express an idea that is just beyond their current grammatical repertoire. The child may be repeating an utterance because we haven't quite grasped the nuance they are expressing. They may re-phrase, or put emphasis on a particular part of the utterance. They may seem unsatisfied either with their current construction, or our understanding of the message: this may be conveyed through their non-verbal communication.

These are clues that we need to help them out with a new grammatical construction that conveys the idea that is in their mind. They may be almost there: the pronoun or the verb construction or the conjunction just needs a tweak. We can model this tweak and monitor the child's reaction. If we've got it, and we've expressed what they wanted to express, they will let us know with an enthusiastic response.

How does stage 4 morph into stages 5 and 6?

Just as we have seen in earlier stages, a child is likely to use a rich mixture of language from different stages. As they acquire more complex language, we see a shift with more language being made up of stages 4, 5 and 6. If they are tired, poorly or dysregulated, we may see more stage 1 and 2 language. When they are alert and better regulated, they may access later stage language.

Towards the end of stage 4, a child is able to produce sentences that include the following:

- All basic pronouns: I, me, my, mine, you, your, yours, we, our, ours, they, their, theirs, them, he, him, him, she, her, hers, it, this, that.

- Basic verb constructions: present tenses with the uninflected verb, e.g. 'I walk' and the present progressive 'I am walking'; irregular and regular past tense 'we ate', 'we danced'; future tense 'I'm going to play'.

- Some auxiliary verbs to modulate meaning: 'we could build it', 'I did see it'.

- Early negatives, e.g. 'it's not blue', 'it's not working'.

- Early question forms, e.g. 'who?' 'what?' 'where?' 'how many?', 'how much?'

Stage 5 is a natural extension of this. We might start to see in our language samples the following stage 5 constructions:

- Pronouns such as 'no one' and 'nobody'.

- Reflexive pronouns such as 'myself', 'ourselves' and 'herself'.

- Modifiers such as 'nothing' and 'none'.

- Auxiliary verbs 'can', 'will', 'may', 'could', 'would', 'should' and 'did'.

- Reversal of auxiliary verbs such as 'do they play?' and 'can I come?'.

- Conjunctions 'but', 'so', 'so that' and 'or'.

Stage 6 is the most sophisticated grammar. We hear sentences that include:

- Pronouns such as 'anybody', 'anyone', 'everybody' and 'everyone'.

- Modifiers such as 'anything', 'everything', 'both', few', 'many', 'first' and 'last'.

- Auxiliary verbs 'must come' and 'shall go'.

- Verbs functioning as nouns (gerund) 'bouncing is fun' and 'I love reading'.

- Uncontracted negatives 'I can not' and 'she has not gone'.

- Subordinate clauses containing the conjunctions 'where', 'when', 'how', 'until', while', 'unless', 'before' and 'after'.

- Reversal of auxiliary 'have': 'has he see you?' and 'have we finished?'.

- Question forms containing 'why?', 'what if?', 'how come?', 'how about?', 'whose?' and 'which?'.

How can we be sure that this is self-generated language?

It can be difficult to know if a sophisticated sentence is a stage 1 gestalt, a stage 2 mitigation, or stage 5 or 6 language. We will look for multiple examples of a particular linguistic structure in our language samples. So for example if they use the conjunction 'but' in several sentences, e.g. 'we went to the post office but it was closed', 'It was my birthday but I was ill', 'I asked for coke but they gave me lemonade', we can be confident that this is self-generated language.

When do we start supporting stage 5 language?

If a child's language sample is showing us that they are over 50% in stage 4, we can start modelling stage 5. Another indication is that they are trying to express more complex ideas than their current stage 4 grammar allows.

Developmental sentence analysis (Laura Lee, 1974)[1]

Laura Lee's Developmental Sentence Analysis (see the previous chapter) allows us to analyse language samples and track grammatical development from stages 4 through to stage 6 of Natural Language Acquisition.

Table 9.2 shows the Developmental Sentence Scoring (DSS) levels against the Natural Language Acquisition stages:

Table 9.2 Quick reference comparing DSS levels with NLA stages

DSS levels	NLA stage
1–3	4
4–6	5
7–8	6

Each DSS level represents grammar that naturally emerges at approximately the same time. Each level provides a foundation for the next level.

It is worth noting that the DSS is based on Analytic Language Processors' language acquisition. With more research, it may become clear that there are differences with Gestalt Language Processors' order of acquisition, but for now, this is the best tool we have.

Just like with previous NLA stages, children will continue to use language from a mix of NLA stages, and therefore will also use a mix of DSS levels. In NLA stage 4 the child will use grammar from levels 1–3 of the DSS (in addition to language from stages 1–3 of NLA). We may also see the odd grammatical construction from later DSS levels, but the child is 'living' in NLA stage 4 and DSS levels 1–3. In stage 5 they will use grammar from DSS levels 4–6 in addition to their established grammar from earlier levels. In stage 6, they will add grammar from DSS levels 7 and 8, moving towards a complete grammar system.

Our language sample analysis changes

When a child is securely in stage 5, the proportions of utterances in each stage become less important than the content of their utterances. We will examine these utterances to see what grammar they have and what grammar they might need.

A structured approach to tracking grammar in stages 4–6

When our language samples show that a child is comfortably using stage 4 grammar, we might print out the DSS (see the handouts section) and highlight the constructions that the child is using, and in a different colour, the constructions that they have yet to acquire in levels 1–3. We might consider throwing in a few of these constructions into our language modelling, if they seem useful for the child. We will do the same when a child is using stage 5 grammar, this time highlighting constructions from DSS levels 4–6 that we might want to model. And the same when a child is moving into stage 6: we will highlight constructions from DSS levels 7 and 8.

We may print out the DSS and highlight the constructions that might be modelled by other adults supporting the child. We will need to stress the continued importance of using this language in as natural a way as possible. When we notice that the child might be trying to express something more complex than their current grammar allows, we add a suggestion for how to convey their intention.

I have created separate handouts (in the handouts section) for each level of DSS as another optional support. This may be less intimidating for families than the whole DSS at once. I have given examples of each grammatical construction.

We're still child-led; we still talk naturally

We still want to be child-led, using this child or young person's enthusiasms and interests in our language modelling. We get our inspiration from knowing a child well.

By now, we may not be the person working directly with the child. We may be providing consultative advice to parents or teaching staff. Therefore we need to stress to others that we continue to be led by the child's interests.

Activity ideas

What follows are some ideas for play that might encourage exploration of grammar.

Pretend play is often a good way to explore the language that a child is using and what further grammar might be helpful. Pretend play with characters in a range of situations will allow for using different pronouns, verb constructions, negatives and question forms.

Depending on a child's enthusiasms, we could use Lego, magnetic tiles, kinetic sand, or art and craft materials. We could draw, take photos, make constructions or try out craft ideas. We can discuss our ideas and potential solutions to problems.

We could look at books: the 'You Choose' series is great for younger children. Books with limited text but rich illustrations stimulate the imagination for older children, for example books by Aaron Becker or Molly Idle. We could watch YouTube 'how to' clips, or those which explore the child's enthusiasms.

Let the individual GLP inspire you. If they love to go into the garden, this may lend itself to such grammatical constructions as 'the peas look ready, but the beans need longer'. If they like being active in the playground we can model 'I can't quite reach, so I'll stand on here'. These everyday life dilemmas and wonderings are often all we need to inspire natural language modelling.

We might feel under pressure at this stage to bring in more traditional Speech and Language Therapy activities: Black Sheep language activities or Blanks Questions, for instance. Whilst the pictures for these resources might sometimes be fun to use, we want to make sure that we are still child-led, still conversational: we are exploring and having fun, rather than eliciting particular language. If the child is not naturally interested in exploring these resources, they are not going to be helpful.

If we think the child is struggling to convey an idea, we can model more complex grammar

If we sense that a child is trying to convey something more complicated than their current grammatical utterance allows, we can offer another way of saying it. So if a child says, 'nobody hasn't got their coats on yet', we might say 'you're right, nobody has their coat on yet'. We will gauge the child's response to this. If we have correctly interpreted the child's intended meaning, we will probably get a sense of this. The conversation will continue, and the child may build on their idea.

Like all language, a child is likely to need to hear a grammatical construction a few times in different contexts before they attempt to use it. Their first experiments may be hesitant, and so we don't want to be too quick to correct them. It is often helpful to acknowledge the meaning first, and perhaps repeating at least part of the utterance before we add to it or change it.

We may need to be more thorough for older GLPs

For a younger child who has been moving through the NLA stages quite quickly and easily, we can take a fairly relaxed approach to supporting stages 5 and 6. We can even trust that they will get there in their own time when they are developmentally ready. Our role may be just to monitor their development through regular language samples, to check that there is movement there.

For an older child who might have been late to Natural Language Acquisition, we might want to be more thorough. We will be considering how dynamic the child's language growth is. If they are creating new language every day we will need a less prescriptive approach, similar to a young child. If their language samples show that they have a restricted variety of stage 5 language, we might focus our modelling on particular constructions and monitor their uptake.

The continuity between spoken and written language

As children become proficient readers, written language becomes an important source for acquiring more complex vocabulary and grammar. Ideally this happens naturally: the child is encouraged to explore books or magazines around their enthusiasms and interests, and as part of this, they encounter written language that is increasingly sophisticated. See Chapter 13 for more information around literacy.

Stages 5 and 6 include academic language

Some grammatical constructions may be explicitly taught in English or used in other subjects (science experiment write-ups offer a rich source of complex grammar, for instance). Schools-based Speech and Language Therapists may work collaboratively with teaching staff so that they can support grammatical development in a classroom context. If a child is struggling to answer a question, either using spoken or written language, a trusted adult may be able to help model the grammar that they need in order to do so more successfully.

This may be the point where Speech and Language Therapy is faded out

Depending on the context of therapy, later stage 5 or stage 6 may mark the point where a child or young person is closed to statutory services. Ideally they will still be supported from indirect support from a Speech and Language Therapist via training or coaching. If a child is to be closed to therapy services, it is important that Speech and Language Therapists provide appropriate resources, and signpost parents or teachers to other supports such as NLA-informed websites or online groups so that those supporting a child or young person can continue to ask questions and seek clarification around continued language acquisition.

Summary of stage 5 and 6 supports

- Continue to prioritise trust and connection.

- Keep connection going by doing 'just enough'.

- Allow silence and space for the child to think and process language.

- Continue to show our authentic selves. We will ponder big ideas together with the child.

- Value and validate all of the child's communication. We don't jump in to correct their experiments with grammar. This is very new to them.

- Embed grammar within play and meaningful conversations. This way we get insight into what the child is needing to express, and how grammar might help.

- Partner with parents to ensure that we are all aware of the child's experiments with grammar, and what the child may be trying to convey with their grammar experiments.

- Talk naturally at least 50% of the time.

- Take regular language samples to track a child's language acquisition, using the DSS to identify constructions that a child is naturally exploring.

- Provide models of particular grammatical constructions where a child seems to need these.

- Use the DSS to guide us in particular grammar that the child has yet to acquire.

- Consider other conversational settings and supporting a child there.

- Keep track of any gaps in grammar or self-expression.

- Add in any constructions that might be particularly helpful or personally significant for this individual.

- Support the merging of spoken and written language: provide opportunities for reading around their enthusiasms, listening to audiobooks or podcasts, accessing technology to search for new information, creating text-based messages and presenting their learning in print.

- Recognise that other aspects of language will continue to grow alongside grammar: e.g. vocabulary, reasoning, different modes of expression.

- Know that in the right circumstances, with attuned communication partners, grammar can continue to grow into late adolescence and early adulthood.

How we track progress in stages 5 and 6

We can look at our language samples and examine them for constructions across the DSS. We will be looking at variety: do they show variety in indefinite and personal pronouns? In verb constructions? In their conjunctions, negatives, interrogative reversals and question forms? We can identify any gaps and aim to model these in natural situations across the day. We may also be considering other aspects of language use, in addition to grammar. We should also consider breadth of vocabulary. We can also look at how the child is using language across contexts, and with whom, and support the generalisation of these skills across settings and situations.

Goals for a stage 5 GLP

A stage 5 goal might be written as:

> *When well-regulated and when supported by a trusted adult, Antoni will use grammatical constructions from levels 4–6 of Laura Lee's Developmental Sentence Analysis (1974). This includes using auxiliary verbs 'can go', 'will go', conjunctions 'but', 'so', 'or' and 'if', and negatives 'can't', 'don't, 'isn't' and 'won't'.*

Goals for a stage 6 GLP

A stage 6 goal might be written as:

> *When well-regulated and when supported by a trusted adult, Antoni will complete his grammar system to incorporate sentences that include subordinate clauses with the words 'where', 'when', 'until', 'before' and 'after', and the question forms 'what if?', 'why?', 'which?' and 'whose?'*

Case study: Antoni

I was carrying out consultative services for Antoni's school, and within a week of reception class starting, Antoni's teacher raised concerns that Antoni was very quiet and did not always appear to understand questions or instructions.

Antoni was bilingual, with an English dad and Polish mum. I met with Antoni's parents, and we discussed his language development so far. He had been a little late in his talking, which his parents thought was related to having been in Covid lockdowns in rural Poland and having very little contact with other children or adults.

Through discussions with his parents, it became apparent that Antoni was likely a gestalt processor. He had an excellent memory for events that had happened a long time ago, including repeating exactly what was said and done in a given location.

With his parents' consent, I carried out initial observation in class, and then saw Antoni individually for a play session in a quieter environment.

Antoni presented as a very gentle, sweet little boy. In the classroom observation where he was sitting with three classmates on the carpet for a maths lesson, he was able to use numicon resources, matching the shapes to number cards for 0–5. He was able to focus on this activity for 5–10 minutes. He presented as eager to please, and perhaps a little anxious.

When I saw Antoni for our play session, he was distracted by the noise of the computer server in the room and looked up at this several times. I was able to take a language sample in this session, as Antoni was eager to talk as we played.

When I analysed the language sample, it looked as though Antoni had lots of flexible stage 3 and 4 language. When I shared this with his parents, his mum felt that perhaps his Polish was not quite as advanced as this. His mum read up about Gestalt Language Processing and knew that she could support him by talking naturally, following his lead and occasionally offering new phrases to match his intentions.

We did not have a Polish equivalent of the DSS to refer to, but Antoni's mum felt fairly confident that she could model a similar level of language complexity, expressing a wide range of grammatical constructions in Polish. For example, different pronouns, verb constructions, negatives and question forms.

Over the next few months, I took two further language samples which showed a steady acquisition of a range of grammatical structures in stage 4. Each time I took a language sample I shared this with Antoni's parents and they provided feedback about his language use in Polish. At one point Antoni's mum expressed concerns about his behaviour at Polish club, as Antoni would avoid interaction and instead move chairs around at the back of the room to create a train. He would then play with his brother on the train, instead of joining the group. We problem-solved this together and wondered if the noise of the sessions were dysregulating for Antoni. Also perhaps he felt a little under pressure to join in and talk. Antoni's mum decided that she would reduce the pressure to join in and allow Antoni to just listen from afar.

By the end of the spring term, my language sample showed that Antoni was entering stage 5 of NLA, with lots of DSS constructions from levels 1 through to 5, and a couple of level 6 constructions. It was clear from the language sample that our job as adults was simply to listen attentively and help Antoni express the more complex thoughts and narratives with a little more grammar than he currently had. By listening carefully, we could co-construct a coherent story, and Antoni could tell us whether we had correctly interpreted what he was trying to convey with his very clear 'nopes' or 'yeahs'!

Two examples of this are shown in Table 9.3. In the first excerpt, Antoni is telling a story about a goose, and in the second he is speculating about the activities and current location of the Easter Bunny. In each of these excerpts I'm supporting Antoni to tell a story: this naturally allows me to use slightly more complex grammar than he currently has.

You will note that I have not scored utterances where Antoni just says, 'yeah' or 'nope'. In stages 4–6 we are scoring grammatical constructions. Utterances that do not contain grammar can be left aside from scoring. They are an essential part of conversation, but not part of our language sample scoring.

Table 9.3 Antoni's language sample

17	Ant	Wow! That's why the goose was in the forest.	DSS 8 (that's why)	6
	Ali	The goose was in the forest?		
18	Ant	Yes.		
19	Ant	Cos it seened something.	DSS 6 (because)	5
	Ali	Oh, it had seen something.		
20	Ant	He seen a person.	DSS 2 (he)	4
	Ali	Oh, was he scared?		
21	Ant	Yep. And he falled in the mud.	DSS 2 (he)	4
	Ali	And did he get all muddy?		
22	Ant	Yeah.		
	Ali	So the goose saw the person and he fell in the mud.		
23	Ant	So . . . so the . . . person . . . and the goose seen him and then he seen him.	DSS 3 (and)	4
	Ali	Did he get a shock?		
24	Ant	yeah.		
	Ali	So sometimes when we get a shock or a surprise, we jump. We jump in surprise.		
25	Ant	Yeah.		
	Ali	Poor goose.		

(Continued)

29	Ant	So he . . . but my mummy had some chocolate from the shops.	DSS 5 (but, so – emerging)	5
	Ali	And has she hidden it high up? On a shelf?		
30	Ant	yes.		3
	Ali	Yes. So we can't eat it before Easter.		
31	Ant	Because it's Easter today.	DSS 6 (because)	5
	Ali	Oh, it's Easter in two weeks.		
32	Ant	yes.		
	Ali	We have to wait a bit longer.		
33	Ant	So the Easter bunny's going to take ages.	DSS 5 (so)	5
	Ali	Yes, the Easter bunny will come in two weeks, which is quite long wait.		
34	Ant	Maybe the Easter bunny's hiding.	DSS 1	4
	Ali	Yeah. Maybe the Easter bunny is sorting out all of the easter eggs, and wrapping them up.		
35	Ant	Maybe the Easter bunny's hiding there?	Pointing to the cupboard DSS 1	4
	Ali	He might be! He might be really busy in the cupboard wrapping easter eggs!		

36	Ant	Cos he's in that door, busy in there.	DSS 6 (because)	5
	Ali	Really busy. Saying 'I need Easter eggs for Antoni! I need Easter eggs for Ali! I need Easter eggs for Antoni's mummy and daddy!		
37	Ant	But, so how we're going to do?	DSS 5 (infinitive complement)	5
	Ali	So what's he going to do? Because he's so busy!		
38	Ant	No, he's not busy. He's having lots of . . . lots of work.	DSS 2 (he)	4
	Ali	Hmm. He's got lots of work to do, but maybe the Easter bunny likes being busy.		
39	Ant	yup.		
	Ali	Cos that's the Easter bunny's job.		
40	Ant	So the Easter bunny's too fat to eat a lot of ice-cream.	DSS 5 (infinitive complement; so)	5
	Ali	Ah. So the Easter bunny just gives out easter eggs to other people. That's very kind.		
41	Ant	Yep. So he's hiding somewhere.	DSS 5 (so)	5

(Continued)

42	Ant	Maybe he's hiding in that corridor?	DSS 2 (he)	4
	Ali	Oh, could be in the corridor, could be in the cupboard . . . he could be in his special Easter bunny hole in the ground.		
43	Ant	Yep.		
	Ali	That nobody knows about.		
44	Ant	But nobody knows about the cupboard.	DSS 5 (but)	5
45	Ant	He can't say anything to us.	DSS 4 (can't)	5
	Ali	We can't find the Easter eggs before Easter. We have to wait.		
46	Ant	We have to wait for two weeks because . . . because . . . I think it's . . . I think it's time to finish.	DSS 6 (because)	5
	Ali	I think it is time to finish. I think you are right. And we're going to have to wait for those eggs.		

Note

1 Lee, L. (1974) *Developmental Sentence Analysis: A Grammatical Assessment Procedure for Speech and Language Clinicians* Northwestern University Press.

Chapter 10

Regulation supports

Ayres sensory integration

Jean Ayres, author of two seminal works on sensory processing[1,2], described sensory processing as the 'organisation of sensation for use'. Our brains have to register, interpret and integrate inputs from the following sensory systems:

- Interoception: information about how our body is feeling; hunger, thirst, temperature, needing the toilet; our state of alertness, our awareness of discomfort or pain in our body; awareness of our emotional state.

- Tactile: the sensations of touch and pressure; the perception of an object's touch qualities, e.g. hard or soft, smooth or rough.

- Vestibular: where our body is in relation to gravity; the perception of speed and direction of movement.

- Proprioception: information about particular parts of the body, e.g. how they are positioned and how they are moving.

- Smell: information about different types of smell, e.g. musty, flowery, pungent.

- Taste: information about different types of taste, e.g. sweet, sour, salty, bitter.

- Visual: information about what we are seeing: the whole picture in terms of positions and depth perception; light, patterns and colours; movement effects.

- Auditory: information about sounds in our environment and the ability to filter these out in relation to other stimuli such as speech; musical qualities of speech, e.g. pitch, rate, volume.

When these inputs are functioning well, they allow a child to:

- Attend to the most important stimuli, e.g. someone speaking.

- Coordinate a response to stimuli, e.g. respond to a person.

- Make postural adjustments, e.g. balance the weight of the torso when sitting.

- Coordinate fine and gross motor movements, e.g. pick up small objects whilst sitting.

- Carry out sequenced motor plans, e.g. walk up stairs.

DOI: 10.4324/9781032717029-10

- Coordinate eyes and hands, e.g. reach for an object.

- Learn about spatial relationships, e.g. navigate a cluttered room, proximity to others.

- Develop a body plan, e.g. know where our limbs are in space at any given time.

- Gain awareness of internal states, e.g. know when we need to use the toilet.

- Make predictions about the world, e.g. predict how an object will move.

- Develop executive function, e.g. decide on the most important action right now.

- Develop bilateral skills for dressing, feeding, using equipment.

- Develop communication and language skills, e.g. vocalise in response to someone.

- Access speech, e.g. reliably use mouth words to express ideas.

When to seek the support from a sensory integration trained therapist

Occupational Therapists, Physiotherapists and Speech and Language Therapists can become sensory integration trained therapists. As such they are able to assess a child's sensory needs and design an individualised programme of support. If a child's sensory needs are impacting on their wellbeing, play, learning or language acquisition, we should signpost them to these services.

The balance of regulation

Regulation might be seen as a continuum (Figure 10.1). We move up and down this continuum throughout the day. Let's say that below 0 is under-stimulated, whilst 1–2 is the feeling of being extremely relaxed and calm, but we don't feel like doing much. From 3–8, we are both relaxed and alert. We are ready for playful learning, experimenting, being creative. We are engaged and energised. If we rev up to 9–10 we are in a state of high excitement: we might be unable to contain the energy in our body and so we need to bounce, spin, squeal or shout. Beyond 10 we have tipped into being overstimulated, overwhelmed, hyper or even frightened. When we are in a state of flight, fright or freeze, we are in this territory. This is also the place of total meltdown.

For optimal language acquisition, we probably want a chid to be in the calm alert zone for much of our session, but it is ok if they move up and down and have 'revved' up moments and calmer moments.

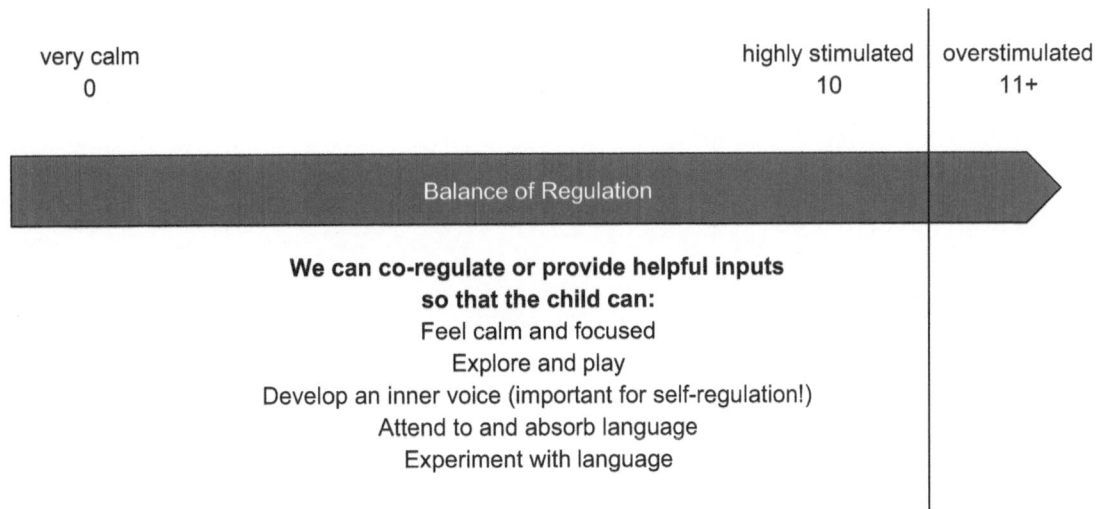

Figure 10.1 The balance of regulation

'The Balance of Regulation' adapted from Cummins (2021)[3]

Co-regulation

We tend to pick up on the 'energy in the room'. If we are with a stressed-out person, we feel that stress. If we are with a deeply chilled person, we become a little more chilled. It is the same for children. We can magnetise them with our energy. If they are entering the room using a high-pitched, loud, staccato voice, then we can be quiet, and when we do talk, we use a deeper, softer, slower, more mellifluous tone. If they are zipping around all over the place, we might offer some regulating rocking movements, linear swinging, and then, when they are still, some deep pressure to their joints. We are slow, predictable, intentional, calm.

A dysregulated child will quickly dysregulate us, unless we can consciously use our emotional regulation strategies or sensory strategies to bring us both back into a state of calm. That's why it is important to be aware of our regulation, minute to minute. Once we know a few sensory strategies, we can regulate ourselves, and at the same time we will be helping to regulate a child. This also works for parents and professionals we are working with: adults will also mirror our energy.

Alerting supports

The following supports are very generalised. We should seek support from a sensory integration trained therapist where possible to personalise supports.

To bring ourselves or others up the regulation continuum, energising and alerting us when we are feeling sleepy and slow, we provide sensory inputs that are:

- Faster.

- Louder.

- Lighter.

- Novel.

Calming supports

To bring ourselves or others down the regulation continuum, calming ourselves when we are feeling jangly and stressed, we provide sensory inputs that are:

- Slower.

- Quieter.

- Predictable.

- Familiar.

Some examples are shown in Table 10.1.

Regulation rhythms within a session

A therapy session will have a rhythm to it. There will be modulation between being calm and relaxed, being well-regulated and being highly energised. An attuned therapist will be able to recognise when a child has had a huge burst of energy and excitement and now needs some quiet time to down-regulate. Often children will do this themselves: they will move away and busy themselves in the furthest corner of the room. This is good: they are learning to self-regulate. By allowing periods of quiet, periods of aloneness, we are supporting regulation.

Tipping into dysregulation

We will not always get it right. When we are getting to know a child (and even with children we know well) we will sometimes accidentally tip them into dysregulation. Our game of chase or our singing of a song will just be a bit too high-energy or go on for too long, and the child will have to release their energy by hitting, biting or scratching.

We don't take this personally. Often a child will be very upset that this happened. We take this as important information: we have a child who is struggling to manage their regulation and who can easily tip into dysregulation. We will need to be sensitive to this, and try to build in down-regulating activity into our sessions. We won't always get it right. We can acknowledge this to the child and anyone else

Table 10.1 Alerting and calming supports

Alerting supports	Calming supports
Using a fast, loud, high-pitched, staccato voice.	Using a slow, quiet, low-pitched, mellifluous voice.
Moving quickly: jumping or skipping in unpredictable ways; playing chase.	Moving slowly: crawling through or under objects; being slowly squished.
Non-linear swinging or spinning; switching direction suddenly; starting and stopping.	Linear swinging; a predictable pace with no sudden changes; preparing for stopping.
Chasing a ball or a balloon that moves in unpredictable ways.	Steady rolling of a weighted ball back and forth in a predictable direction.
Music with a jumpy, unpredictable rhythm and changing tempos, e.g. 'Sleeping Bunnies'.	Music with a steady, predictable pace and rhythm, e.g. 'Row Your Boat' sung slowly.
Being tickled; light touch; 'Round and Round the Garden' on the palm of the hand, or 'This Little Piggy' on the toes.	Deep pressure to the joints in a predictable sequence; being squished slowly with the same words being used each time.
Toys which move in unpredictable ways: balloons, pump-up rockets, toys with pop-up parts.	Toys which are heavy and move in predictable ways: wooden blocks, lining up, completing a sequence.

in the room. We don't have to be perfect, and it is helpful to show that we too are learning.

Tuning in to our own regulation

Becoming aware of our own state of regulation is helpful, and we can get better at it the more we practice. We might check in with ourselves before seeing a child. Many techniques of mindfulness are helpful here, for example carrying out a body scan, moving through parts of our body in turn. If something feels 'off' we might do a quick audit:

- Am I hungry or thirsty?

- Am I too hot or cold?

- Is my clothing uncomfortable?

- Is anything in this environment causing me discomfort? For example, lighting, noise, seating.

- Am I tired? Revved up? Stressed about something?

We can add to this list, depending on what we learn about ourselves from regular practice. For example, we may be prone to low blood sugar, or headaches from too bright lighting.

Quick regulation hacks

Regulation supports are highly personal, but some quick tricks we can try to bring ourselves into a state of regulation include:

- Noticing three things we can see, three things we can hear, three things that we can feel.

- Feeling the soles of our feet (calming) or the tips of our fingers (energising).

- Breathing slowly for ten breaths, consciously extending the exhale.

Emotional regulation

Emotional dysregulation occurs when a person feels that others are not 'getting them'. Something has happened that has caused distress. If another person in the room picks up on this distress, and shows empathy and concern, or takes steps to alleviate our distress, then we are more likely to calm. We feel understood, 'seen' and nurtured. If that does not happen, we will continue in our dysregulated state. If we continue to feel misunderstood, not seen, ignored or resisted, we will likely tip into meltdown. That's not to say that we always have to 'give in' to a child: we can provide safe boundaries, but we do this with empathy and understanding. We acknowledge their frustration or longing. We use language that is conciliatory and inclusive, e.g. 'We can't go up there. I wish we could'. If they are in total meltdown, we don't use any language. We offer calm, concerned presence, probably from a distance, and wait for them to come back down.

Development of an inner voice

The development of an inner voice is likely to be as important for regulation as it is for language acquisition. When we provide calm and silence, we allow space and time for a child to use their inner voice. When we provide well-timed, sensitive language models for self-advocacy and expressing sensory needs, we offer the language of a helpful inner voice that a child may later draw on in order to self-regulate. This is one of the reasons that we prioritise the communication intentions of 'expressing joy', 'expressing sensory needs', 'self-advocacy' and 'protesting'. We are aiming to model a possible future soundtrack for a child's inner voice.

Neurodivergent children may struggle with interoception

Neurodivergent adults tell us that they struggle to recognise their body signals for hunger, thirst, cold, heat, digestive discomfort and so on. They are more likely to experience gut issues, sleep disorders, eating disorders, headaches and migraines. It is unclear whether this is due to neurodivergence itself or a consequence of living in a world that prioritises the neurotypical experience. Chronic dysregulation will not help a person develop good interoception. If we don't help autistic children to develop bodily autonomy and give them access to regulatory supports, e.g. being allowed to stim, then they will not learn about their internal states and their innate ability to ease bodily discomfort.

There is a close relationship between sensory integration and emotional regulation

Sensory integration is inextricably linked with emotional regulation. If we are experiencing unpredictable or unpleasant sensory inputs, if we are operating in a world which is constantly confusing or disorientating because of its sensory complexity, then we will be emotionally dysregulated. We may be overwhelmed or distressed or in a state of fight, flight or freeze for much of our time.

Think of a time when one of your sensory systems was not working optimally. You couldn't find your glasses, you had blocked ears, you were sunburnt or had itchy skin, or your sense of smell and taste were off. How was your emotional regulation at that time?

If a child is frequently distressed, if they are acting out or withdrawing, if they are fearful or aggressive in certain environments, then we probably need to consider their sensory needs and potential medical issues.

Problem-solving around sensory needs

Regulation supports are individual. The activities that a child seeks out or avoids may provide us with clues as to what they may need in order to feel regulated. In Table 10.2 are some examples of what a child is doing, why they might be doing this and what we might provide to further support them.

Table 10.2 Problem-solving around sensory needs

What the child is doing	Why the child seeks this	What we might provide
Running, jumping, spinning	May be craving vestibular and proprioceptive stimulation.	Linear swinging. Bouncing on a trampoline or therapy ball. Wearing a tight Lycra suit and pushing against it.
Crashing, bumping, clinging	May be craving stronger tactile, vestibular and proprioceptive stimulation.	Check for ear infection. Jumping onto crash-pads, being squashed between cushions, on a peanut ball, or rolled in a blanket. Push-ups against the wall. Heavy work, like pushing a wheelbarrow or carrying a heavy backpack. Deep pressure squeezes to joints.
Struggles to sit still	May be craving vestibular and proprioceptive input to feel where they are in space. May have weak core stability.	Provide vestibular and proprioceptive input before a short period of sitting still. Use a chair that allows the child to rock, e.g. Zuma chair. Or use a weighted lap cushion, textured seat pad or therapy bands tied to legs of chair to allow some rocking or proprioceptive feedback for legs. Build core strength with climbing, reaching, hanging from bars, sitting or rolling on peanut or therapy ball.
Biting or teeth-grinding	May be trying to stabilise the body in order to feel calm.	Chewy tubes and chewable necklaces or bracelets: a range of resistance levels are available. Minimise exposure to dysregulating inputs. Deep pressure to provide stability.

What the child is doing	Why the child seeks this	What we might provide
Flapping or flicking fingers	May be trying to block out other stimuli or 'reset' by focusing on something within their control. Often a response to being rushed by another person.	Allow them to stim! Minimise exposure to dysregulating inputs. Give the person time to complete an activity before rushing into the next.
Eating non-edible items	May be craving smell, taste or tactile stimulation.	Vibrating toys, including a vibrating toothbrush. Crunchy and chewy foods with a strong taste.
Takes off clothes	May be very sensitive to labels or seams, or particular fabrics.	Experiment with seamless clothing with no labels, and with very soft textures. Allow the child to choose their own clothing.
Avoids car rides or imposed movements	May be very sensitive to vestibular input.	Drive forwards out of driveway rather than reversing. Take corners slowly. Warn of any upcoming turns or stops.
Avoids stairs or walking on uneven surfaces	May experience gravitational insecurity. May be sensitive to heights and feeling unbalanced.	Gradual exposure to heights and vestibular activities. Singing 'Row Your Boat' and 'Rock Your Boat' whilst being held may be a good first step. Make rocking movements very predictable, accompanied by song or a phrase. Partners being sensitive to signs to stop.

(Continued)

What the child is doing	Why the child seeks this	What we might provide
Avoids wet or messy play	May have extremely sensitive touch receptors in the hands so that changes in temperature, wetness or stickiness is overwhelming or painful.	Deep pressure and massage is likely to be more pleasant than light touch. Wash hands using deep pressure squeezes to the finger joints. Offer dry sensory play, e.g. dry rice, beans. Offer theraputty or playdough.
Sensitivity to sudden sounds	May have extremely sensitive hearing. May be sensitive to certain frequencies or voice qualities.	Help the child to feel in control of their own environment and choose a quiet space when needed. Use ear defenders or ear plugs in noisy environments. Prepare for any sudden loud noises, e.g. hand-driers. Chewy tubes may help to provide competing sensory input in order to dull the sound.

This is not a prescription for any one child: a sensory integration trained therapist will be able to advise on the specific needs of a child. This is especially important where there is a history of trauma.

Movement and speech

Children often become more vocal when they are engaged in a vestibular activity like jumping, running, tumbling, swinging or bouncing. Some children may need to get quite hyped up before they can access their voice. If this is the case, we may need to think about bringing them down the regulation scale again at the end of our session.

Children are more likely to take deep belly breaths when they are engaged in movement. If they are leaning over a therapy ball or a rubber tyre swing, the belly breaths are likely to be deeper, because there is compression and release in the abdomen.

When a child is well-regulated, they are more likely to be able to organise their body for movement patterns (praxis). The more regulation they experience, the better able they are to establish movement patterns in their body, and for speech.

Breath support for speech

Speech is dependent on breath support. For good breath support, we need core stability and strength. Activities which stimulate the vestibular system, and require a child to stabilise their bodies, are also likely to build core strength. So when we gently rock a child on a therapy ball, we are likely helping them establish core strength which will ultimately help their breath support for speech.

Joyful vocalisation

Furthermore, these movements are often delightful and exciting to a child (we will have to grade the degree of movement: it is a fine line between excitement and overstimulation or fear). This will often lead to spontaneous joyful noises like 'wee!', 'woo!' or giggling. These sounds are important because the child is switching their voice on and off (getting started and stopping a movement pattern can often be the most challenging). The child is learning to sustain their voice for open vowels and semivowels. Laughter requires deep belly breaths and helps to initiate consonant-vowel strings, e.g. 'hahaha!'

Core strength

Core strength also comes from moving from sitting to a quadruped position on hands and knees, and back again. Leaning from side to side and reaching in a quadruped position will further develop core stability. Any activity on the floor with lots of pieces of toys spread out in front of us will naturally encourage these movements. Crawling through a pop-up tunnel or under a table will also help.

Stimming and regulation

Many neurodivergent adults tell us that they have spent years trying to mask their sensory and movement needs, in order to look neurotypical. It has not been uncommon in schools and therapy to require a child to sit quietly, to still their bodies and to suppress their natural need to movement. The need for movement is sometimes called 'stimming', and can take the form of jiggling, bouncing, flapping or flicking fingers, or fiddling with objects.

Neurodivergent individuals often need to move or to stim in order to stay regulated, and therefore in order to attend, to process and to learn. We need to provide for this in our therapy sessions. We can provide fidget toys, and give unrestricted access to movement. Bouncing and wriggling is good for us all in order to stay focused and well.

We should not use reward charts or 'I'm working towards' charts that withhold sensory supports. These are training an autistic child to mask their needs.

The difference between a tantrum and a meltdown

Meltdowns are triggered by emotional dysregulation, sensory overload fatigue or illness. They are not goal-oriented. A meltdown is not being used as a way to get someone else to do something.

A tantrum is different. It is about trying to get something or achieving a particular result. For example, 'I want the sweets from your bag, and I'm going to sit here and cry and kick until I get them'. Children having tantrums check to see if their behaviour is working. If they are ignored, they might escalate, or give up. Reasoning or bargaining can help.

During a tantrum, our protective mechanisms are intact and we are not likely to hurt ourselves. We are in control, and we are trying to manipulate another person. If the goal is accomplished, our tantrum will stop.

In a meltdown there's no goal; the child is just completely overloaded. They can't process language. Reasoning or bargaining won't work. Using behavioural methods is likely to create further stress, and to traumatise them.

For a child experiencing a meltdown, they need us to:

- Make the space safe for them. Their own ability to keep their bodies safe is currently impaired. We remove ourselves and others from the immediate space, we remove any items that may cause harm, and if possible, we get them to a familiar safe space.

- Use minimal language. We use a deep, slow, quiet, soothing voice to say, 'it's ok' or 'I'm here'. We use affirming, supportive language.

- Offer a safe routine or a down-regulating activity to bring the person into a regulated state. The child may have a comforting toy or sensory activity that helps with this.

- Show empathy and understanding. We don't hold grudges about what might have happened. We understand that they will be upset about the episode.

- Consider the possible influence of illness, fatigue or an undiagnosed chronic medical condition like gastrointestinal distress or migraine.

- Learn about their sensory needs, to avoid meltdowns in the future. We need to be proactive about a child's sensory needs, providing access to regulatory supports so that meltdowns are avoided.

- Listen to parents. They may be dealing with their child's meltdowns at the end of the school day if the school environment is not providing for a child's sensory needs. Too often parents' concerns are dismissed. We need to take parents' reports of meltdowns seriously, because this is a health and wellbeing, and ultimately, a safeguarding concern.

Speech fails when a child is dysregulated

We know from autistic adults that their speech is not always accessible to them. This is more likely to happen the more dysregulated they are. Therefore it is vital for us to advocate for meeting the sensory needs of autistic children.

If an autistic child is dysregulated for a third of the day, this is a third of the day that they are unable to communicate effectively. This will hugely affect their language acquisition. One of the best things we can do as their Speech and Language Therapist is to educate caregivers and educators about the need to meet the sensory and movement needs of autistic children.

Personal regulation supports

Objects or pictures personal to the child may be regulating for them. We are all familiar with 'transitional objects' which help young children transition from a familiar place to an unfamiliar place. These may serve autistic children throughout childhood and into adulthood. Autistic adults report that sometimes objects can be an immense comfort and source of regulation in times of stress. Consider photos or pictures or favourite activities too as personal regulation supports. Many autistic people find counting or reciting rote scripts regulating.

Time spent in nature; time spent with animals

Time spent in nature[4] and time spent with animals[5,6] are consistently reported as being highly regulating for autistic people. The predictable patterns and soothing sounds in nature and the companionship and connection from animals are regulating from both a sensory and emotional perspective.

Universal design and reasonable adjustments in school (and beyond)

Our world is very much designed for neurotypicals. With increasing awareness of neurodiversity, we hope that this is changing. What is vital for autistic people is often highly beneficial for neurotypical people. For instance we all benefit from time outdoors, access to quiet spaces, less cluttered spaces and softer lighting.[7]

If a school building has not been designed with neurodiversity in mind, there are reasonable adjustments that can be made. This includes (but is not restricted to):

- Being able to choose where we sit in a room so that adverse sensory inputs are minimised.

- Being able to get up and move freely, within lessons as well as between lessons.

- Having unrestricted access to fidget toys; being able to openly stim.

- Access to weighted blankets or clothing.

- Seating that allows wobbling and rocking.

- Opportunities to carry out 'heavy work', e.g. carrying a heavy backpack, handing out equipment.

- Access to outdoor space at regular intervals during the day.

- Unrestricted access to a quiet space.

- Sensory circuits or a sensory diet designed by an OT trained in sensory integration.

- A reduced school timetable.

- Some degree of remote learning.

- Positive attitudes to neurodiversity within the learning environment.

These reasonable adjustments are all geared towards making everyday life bearable for a neurodivergent child. We are looking to prevent meltdowns and prevent autistic burnout. We are looking to support a child to learn and thrive in school, in future employment, in our communities and in society. We have a long way to go, but the steps are very achievable.

Notes

1 Ayres, J. (1973) *Sensory Integration and Learning Disorders* Western Psychological Services.
2 Ayres, J. (1979) *Sensory Integration and the Child* Western Psychological Services.
3 Cummins, K. (2021) *Why Mutual Face Watching Matters: Reinforcing Regulation, Wellbeing, Communication and Learning Through Video* J&R Press.

4 Friedman, S., Noble, R., Archer, S., Gibson, J. & Hughes, H. (2023) 'Respite and connection: Autistic adults' reflections upon nature and well-being during the Covid-19 pandemic' *Autism* 27(8), 2483–2495.

5 Hwang, Y. I. J., Foley, K. R. & Trollor, J. N. (2017, December) 'Aging well on the autism spectrum: The perspectives of autistic adults and carers' *International Psychogeriatrics* 29(12).

6 Siewertsen, C. M., French, E. D. & Teramoto, M. (2015, Spring) 'Autism spectrum disorder and pet therapy' *Advances in Mind Body Medicine* 29(2), 22–25.

7 For more information about Universal Design concepts see Zwilling, M. & Levy, B. R. (2022) 'How well environmental design is and can be suited to people with Autism Spectrum Disorder (ASD): A natural language processing analysis' *International Journal of Environmental Research and Public Health* 19(9), 5037.

Chapter 11

GLP and access to speech

Non-speaking, minimally speaking, unreliably speaking

These terms are all used to describe a child or adult who is likely to have internal language that is not reflected in their speech output. 'Non-speaking' would describe an individual who does not speak at all; 'minimally speaking' would describe a person who uses very little speech (a few words or phrases); 'unreliably speaking' describes someone who can speak sometimes, but there are also times when they cannot access speech. This may be due to dysregulation, fatigue, illness or other reasons.

Prevalence of dyspraxia in autism

There is evidence to suggest that between 25% and 30% of autistic people are non-speaking or minimally speaking.[1] This may be due to deep dyspraxia or apraxia of speech, whereby it is very hard for the person to coordinate their breathing, phonation, resonance and articulation in order to produce speech-like sounds.

Families of non-speaking autistic people often report that once in a while, they will hear a perfectly formed phrase or word. It is such a rare thing that communication partners may doubt that it really happened. Attempts from communication partners to get the person to repeat the utterance are usually fruitless: it is a feature of dyspraxia that the more we try to repeat a motor pattern, the harder it is.

The role of AAC

If a child is dyspraxic, we probably want to introduce AAC (Augmentative and Alternative Communication) to add to their communication repertoire. In my experience, all forms of AAC, but especially voice-output AAC help to increase a child's vocalisations. So please read this chapter in conjunction with the chapter about AAC. I strongly suggest a two-pronged approach: work on access to speech using the suggestions in this chapter and also work on AAC using the suggestions in the following chapter.

Presume competence; respect human dignity

One of the most powerful things we can do as a Speech and Language Therapist (or as a communication partner) is to presume competence. We assume that the

DOI: 10.4324/9781032717029-11

autistic person understands everything. They understand our every non-verbal and spoken message to them, to the people around them. We don't talk about them as though they are not in the room. We use language which is respectful and honours their unique contribution to the world.

Autistic advocate Julia Bascom[2] reminds us that we don't presume competence because the child might not have an intellectual disability. We presume competence because we respect human dignity for all human beings.

If we think we heard a minimally speaking child say a word or phrase, we did. If it was a vowel sound or syllable structure which could have been the word 'again' or the phrase 'that one', we assume that it was, and we repeat it. This, in my experience, makes it far more likely that we will hear other communication attempts. Success breeds success. The autistic person gets the message from us that we are listening, and that it is worth their while in attempting communication.

Are they really non-speaking?

We have probably all had experiences where a child has been described as a non-speaker (or non-verbal, to use an outdated and inaccurate term), only for us to find that they are attempting words and phrases, but that these are not being recognised by communication partners.

We are lucky as Speech and Language Therapists to be able to recognise speech when it occurs. We have experience of hearing and interpreting immature phonology, imprecise articulation and dyspraxic speech: our ears are primed for it. When speech takes the form of open vowels, imprecise consonants or reduplicated syllable structures, we know that this is early speech, and that it is important. We know that singing is also speech. Other adults may initially surprised by what we can hear, but then find that they quickly become more adept themselves at listening out for these, just because they are expecting them. When we presume competence, we become better listeners: we hear quiet speech where there is very little breath support; we notice that the open vowel sound is in fact a word.

Are they really dyspraxic?

We will need to get to know a child and develop their trust before we can assess whether they are dyspraxic, or whether they have undeveloped potential with speech. If it is the latter, it may be that they gave up attempting speech because communication partners were not tuned in. If we can prime communication partners to expect speech and listen carefully, this may be enough to get things going again.

The child may naturally start to experiment more and achieve success with finding their voice.

We also need to consider sensory integration and regulation. We may need to help a child to 'rev up' to access their speech, or we may need to help them be more relaxed in order to access their speech. Working with an Occupational Therapist trained in sensory integration may be invaluable here.

Verbal dyspraxia may be mild, moderate or severe. A milder case may involve vowel and consonant errors and problems with multisyllabic words or longer sentences. A more severe case may involve breath support and phonation, so that voice cannot get started in the first place. There may be difficulties with sustaining airflow and phonation, achieving a constant volume or pitch, and controlling nasal versus oral resonance. It may be that many of our non-speaking GLPs are experiencing a severe form of dyspraxia where they can't reliably achieve the breath support for phonation.

What needs to be in place before speech can develop?

It is worth going back to basics here. Before we get to accurate articulation we need:

- Voice requires breath. For sustained phonation, we need good breath support. For good breath support and phonation we need:

- Core stability so that we can maintain the breath support for phonation regardless of our body position.

- Sensory integration of our proprioceptive, vestibular and auditory systems so that we can monitor what we are doing with our vocal tract to achieve reliable voice.

- The motor pattern to be able to reliably start and stop and sustain the motor plan of breathing and phonation.

Sensory integration and movement

Sensory integration and movement are key pieces when we are thinking about speech praxis. We cannot have jaw stability until we have worked on core stability. Our auditory system is inextricably linked to our vestibular system. Stimulating one will stimulate the other.

Core stability and strength

Physiotherapists and Occupational Therapists will always think about proximal stability for distal mobility. This means that the core must be stable in order for limbs to work more accurately.

The core must be strong in order for us to access voice. The core gets strong through movement: running, jumping, climbing, reaching, leaning, pushing off from stable objects like the floor, wall or furniture, moving against resistance, pushing, pulling and other heavy work, and stabilising our bodies against gravity as we rock, roll, swing or spin.

So we cannot sit a child at a small table and expect their voice to magically work. We need to get them moving.

Joy allows us to access our voice

Movement is also important because it is joyful. When a child is being swung in a blanket, or lifted high up and 'dropped' by an adult, when they are held at the waist and spun around, when they are being squashed by a peanut ball, they are likely to gasp and take a deep breath. This may lead to spontaneous bursts of laughter, or delighted squeals and yells. Movement allows us to unintentionally access our voice.

A hierarchy of supports

In her article, When Speech Gets Stuck,[3] Marge Blanc lays out an eight-point hierarchy of support that we can use for non-speaking autistic children to help them to naturally access their voice. She emphasises that these are not 'exercises': they are just spontaneous fun activities, which accidentally give rise to voice production.

Just like in the whole NLA framework, we want natural development to occur. There is no imitation, no elicitation, no teaching. If we teach splinter skills we risk them never being generalised into spontaneous speech. We create the conditions that will likely lead to spontaneous development. As always, this is child-led and play-based, with a heavy sprinkling of movement!

We will want the child's family to be providing these supports every day: whatever the level we are at, we will be suggesting activities that the family can carry out little and often. We start from where the child is at: if they don't access their voice at all, we start at level 1 and move up from there. If they are already producing voice reliably when they are laughing, shouting, humming and singing, then we start at level 3.

There are no guarantees with this protocol. However, just moving a child from one level to the next has a huge impact. A child who can reliably vocalise is seen as more communicatively competent by a wider range of communication partners. The ability to vocalise is hugely helpful for a child to signal that they have something to say. When combined with a robust AAC system, their access to communication has improved dramatically.

Level 1: deep breathing

We want to carry out any activity that results in the child getting out of breath, because then they will be using deep belly breathing (also known as abdominal breathing). Running at speed, playing chase, jumping on a bed or trampoline, bouncing on a therapy ball, leaning over a peanut ball, being squished, leaning over a tyre swing, engaging in heavy work, pushing or pulling against resistance . . . these are all likely to lead to deep breathing. This level of support will naturally lead into . . .

Level 2: voice production

We need to find a physical activity that the child finds utterly delightful. It may be being squished, being tickled or dancing to their favourite song. It might be a YouTube clip they find hilarious. It might be swinging, spinning or sliding. It might be climbing up high and jumping down. It might be being swung in a blanket.

People games are important here. Playing monsters or zombies whilst trying to catch the child might lead to squeals and shrieks. Also songs and games with contrast of quiet followed by raucous noise: 'sleeping bunnies' for example, or playing 'sleeping tigers'.

Toys might play a part: blowing up a balloon and letting it go, wind-up toys, toys that jump or spin, rolling cars down a gutter pipe. Noise generates noise, so banging on drums or pounding the keys of a piano often lead to spontaneous vocalisation. Humming into a whistle or singing into a balloon allows a child to 'feel' their voice.

We want to spend time in this stage so that the child can reliably switch the voice on and off, sustain phonation and begin to spontaneously explore variations in volume and pitch. Which leads us into . . .

Level 3: intonation

We will want to listen out for intonation contours in the child's vocalisations. They may spontaneously use these contours in different games. Some games generate high-pitched squealing, e.g. sliding, spinning, screaming, squealing in surprise. Other games generate deep roars and growls, e.g. monsters, squishing games, tug-of-war, pushing or pulling heavy objects.

At this stage, we can listen out for any intonational contours in the child's spontaneous communication. Are we hearing 'uh-oh', 'huh?', 'doh!' and 'wow!' type contours? We can model these with the natural disasters and surprises and confusions of everyday life.

Songs can be very useful here, especially 'Old Macdonald' with its 'ee-ay-ee-ay-oh'. The scream in 'Row Your Boat' or an 'ow' in 'Five Little Monkeys' might be fun.

Speech Pathologist Corrine Zmoos teaches us that autistic children often have perfect pitch: it is worth us learning about intervals of an octave, fourths or fifths, so that we can use these in our songs and phrases with children. If they find our intervals pleasing, they are more likely to join in.

Level 4: stopping and starting

This is a big one for dyspraxic children. We want to encourage them to be able to control the onset of their voice, and to be able to turn it off.

Because the hardest part of initiating voice is getting it started, Marge Blanc suggests that we might sneak a word into their laughter, e.g. 'ha ha hi!' They are already vocalising, but we are encouraging them to change it. We might also shape a squeal into a word, e.g. 'aaaaah-weee!' or 'oh . . . woah!'

The first time a child does this is likely to be an accident, and they will be unable to replicate it. We need to be patient. We know that they can do it, and it will appear again, but we can't force it. We can just set up the conditions for it to reappear. The conditions are, as always, movement, laughter and fun.

As the child gets more experience at this level, they may then be able to reliably produce sounds like 'wee!' and 'wow' and 'yeah'.

Level 5: vowel sounds

Vowel sounds have of course been appearing in earlier levels. Now we will bring out toys and books and songs which are likely to build a repertoire of vowel sounds, including diphthongs and triphthongs. 'Old Macdonald' will be important here, along with any other songs and games that lend themselves to making vowel sounds. Monkeys can say 'ooh-ooh-ohh', and mice might say 'ee-ee-ee'.

We could have a naughty toy where we have to yell 'oy' or an accident-prone toy who yells 'ow'. We might tend to babies or soft toys with soothing 'ah' sounds. We might play matching games and deliberately make bad matches with an 'uh-oh'. We might look in box or bag and exclaim 'oooooh!'

Level 6: consonant sounds

We do not want to teach splinter skills of imitation at this level, and so we want to integrate this with play and exploration. Rhythm and timing are as important as accurate speech sound production, and so the first stage of this will probably be tapping out rhythms and using musical instruments in copying games. This might naturally lead to adding our voices to the cacophony!

We might clap and stamp out rhythms of familiar songs, letting go of the words and simply humming or using a vowel sound. We know that the semi-vowels are a bridge between vowel and consonant, so maybe we will use sounds like 'ayayayayay' and 'oowoowoowoo' first.

Animal and vehicle sounds are useful at this level. We can have lots of fun with 'moo', 'neigh', 'bah' and so on. Imitating household implements like the hoover, dishwasher and coffee machine might be appealing to some children. Songs with fun sounds like 'Wheels on the Bus' and 'This Is the Way the Ladies Ride' encourage sound-making, and the movement will also help. 'I Am the Music Man' offers a range of fun sounds to imitate. Sandra Boynton's books *Moo Baa La la la* and *The Going to Bed Book* are wonderful for fun sounds.

Level 7: syllables

Fun strings of babble come in now. We might start with reduplicated babble sounds, e.g. 'no-no-no-no!' (children often love being able to tell an adult 'no'), noisy animals 'ba-ba-ba' and 'moo-moo-moo'. Some children might find short vowels easier, e.g. 'pop-pop-pop' and others might be able to manage long vowels 'poo-poo-poo'.

The ambulance sound 'nee-nar' can introduce a vowel variation. The cat sound 'miaow' involves a vowel slide.

We are not trying to elicit sound, but explore them through play. We can say 'mmm' and 'yum' and 'yuck' with food play. We can use 'wah wah' with a baby, or 'Rah! Rah!' with a monster or a dinosaur.

Children tend to love the dramatic sounds of sneezing 'achoo!', and comedy coughs. If we can bring it into a people game, all the better. 'Tah dah!' might accompany us pulling an item out of a bag. We might try games like 'I see you!' or 'peekaboo!'

Level 8: refinement of speech sounds

Throughout this process we have been modelling potential stage 1 gestalts, and some of these may now be being used by the child. We want to tune into the intonation pattern so that when the consonants are not consistent or clear, we still recognise the gestalt.

At this point we may consider using techniques from other therapy approaches, such as DTTC (Dynamic Temporal and Tactile Cueing). Since both use functional words and phrases, these might be the same gestalts that we are modelling. As much as possible we want this therapy to be child-led and play-based, in line with the wider NLA approach. We may use an advocacy tool such as 'Talking Mats'[4] to find out the child's priorities in terms of acquiring speech alongside other modalities.

Throughout this process we also will be using AAC with the child. We know from autistic adults that AAC continues to be an important option for communication, particularly in times of dysregulation or fatigue. The next chapter will focus on all things AAC.

Notes

1 Brignell, A., Chenausky, K. V., Song, H., Zhu, J., Suo, C. & Morgan, A. T. (2018, November 5) 'Communication interventions for autism spectrum disorder in minimally verbal children' *Cochrane Database of Systematic Review* 11.
2 Bascom, J. (2014) 'Dangerous assumptions' *Just Stimming Blogpost* https://juststimming.wordpress.com/category/communication/
3 Blanc, M. (2004) 'When speech gets stuck: A hierarchy of practical supports for dyspraxia in children with ASD' *Autism and Asperger's Digest*, September–October.
4 See Talkingmats.com

Chapter 12

GLP and AAC (Augmentative and Alternative Communication)

When might a child need AAC?

A child who is not readily accessing their voice and acquiring spoken words and phrases is a good candidate for AAC.

Children typically start producing their first words and phrases in their second year, at around 12–15 months. Before that they will have gone through stages of cooing (open vowel sounds) and babbling (repeated syllables consisting of consonant and vowel sounds, e.g. 'bababa' and 'bagabama').

If a child is not vocalising at all, then consider that dyspraxia may be an element (see the previous chapter). We will want to support them to develop a more reliable voice, and at the same time we will want to support them with AAC.

There are no prerequisite skills needed before we introduce a child to AAC. We assume competence: that they want to connect and that they want to communicate. We also presume a child's potential to acquire AAC skills. They will not be able to do this until they have had exposure to AAC for a period of time. Our role is to support those around the child to model language using AAC in everyday situations and play, in the way that language modelling has been described throughout this book. We're just offering an additional mode of communication.

Multi-modal communication

We want children to be multi-modal communicators. This includes them using their voice, their face, their body posture and movements, gestures or signs, and paper-based or technology-based AAC.

We will never prompt a child to 'tell us again with AAC'. It is a child's right to choose their mode of communication. If they've already told us non-verbally, they don't need to repeat the same message using their AAC.

Multi-modal communication may be highly creative and unique

GLPs may be communicating with us in ways that we have not, until now, recognised. Consider the arrangement of treasured objects. Consider the colour

DOI: 10.4324/9781032717029-12

sequences that they repeat or play with. Consider what they gaze at through their hands. These are all opportunities for us to connect with them, and validate their modes of expression. Play schemas such as emptying or filling containers, shuffling objects, letting objects fall and bounce, are potentially ways of connecting with another person, so long as that person is receptive.

We want to honour this child's chosen modes of communication, and we may experiment with incorporating this into an AAC system. This may involve capturing images of their creations. For children who like to look at scenes from unusual angles, we may give them access to a camera, and see what they choose to capture. If they love to watch certain visual effects over and over, e.g. pouring water, watching coloured lights, breaking up coloured chalk, we may want to experiment with using this in their AAC system, either with a static picture in a visual scene (read more about this later in the chapter), or if the AAC system allows, an embedded video or a link to a video.

The AAC users themselves are our creative partners in an exploration of what works (and doesn't work) for them. Their responses to our ideas will be key in whether we pursue this line of thought or not.

Recognising that the child is a competent communicator

Introducing AAC to a child results in increased communication skills in other modalities, including in speech.[1] This may be as much due to communication partners as any change in the child. Communication partners are suddenly viewing the child as a communicator. As such, they listen more, and they notice more. This results in the child feeling seen, heard and recognised as a communicator. They reveal more of themselves and their communication. They have communication success: those around them recognise that their subtle change of breathing rate is important; it indicates excitement and engagement. The communication partner models 'let's do that again!' The child's facial expressions are recognised as communicative: 'that's disgusting. Take it away'. Their vocalisations are suddenly heard, possibly because the communication partners are listening, and possibly because the child is gaining in confidence that the world will listen.

Signs that an AAC user is a GLP

So if we know that 25–30% of autistic children are non-speaking or minimally speaking,[2] it is possible that they do not produce enough speech for us to identify that they are using echolalia to communicate. Some children may only be able to access their voices once in a while. How are we going to know whether they are a GLP or ALP?

Let's look back for a moment at Chapter 2 and the signs that a child might be a GLP.

- The child uses long strings of babble-like utterances, often unintelligible, perhaps with one or two recognisable words within them.

- The child marks the number of syllables in a phrase, but the words are not clear.

- The utterances follow distinct intonational patterns. The phrase is said with the same intonation pattern each time.

- The utterance may include certain body movements or gestures, e.g. spreading arms out wide, jumping.

- There may be a distinct voice quality or an accent, which has been retained from the original sound source.

- The child responds positively to music, songs and rhymes, more so than single words in shared play routines.

- The child likes watching, rewinding and rewatching the same video clips on YouTube or other media sources.

- The child seems to be quoting dialogue from video clips, tv or film. Again, the individual words are unclear, but the intonation pattern is there.

- The child seems to particularly love phrases that are rich in emotional meaning. They will be spoken emphatically to convey strong emotions.

- The child may use a gestalt phrase to make an association between a past experience and what is happening now. There is something about the current situation that reminds them of when they first heard their phrase.

- The child may be highly unintelligible, only using open vocalisations with no consonants. They may hum the tune of songs, scripts, phrases or words.

- A non-speaking child may reveal their gestalt tendencies by showing gestalt cognitive processing: they may act out gestalts through body movements, or expect a particular experience to unfold in exactly the same way each time, including extraneous parts that were only present in their first experience.

- The child might love sets of items, e.g. the whole alphabet, all the pieces of a puzzle or components of a building set. They do not like these being broken up or disrupted by adult suggestions (at least in stage 1. In stage 2, this begins to be more acceptable.).

- The child likes to complete a routine or a task, and does not like being interrupted mid-flow. Again this is likely to become more flexible as they move through NLA stages.

- The child needs structure and predictability in their routines.

- At an earlier stage in development, they used echolalia, but have since become minimally or non-speaking. They may whisper their gestalts, use only character voices, or even have internalised this language, and it is now not possible for us to hear it.

- The child has not responded to traditional SLT advice. The copy-and-add strategy of copying back what they have said and adding a word does not seem to work for them.

Robust AAC (for Analytic Language Processors)

Almost all AAC solutions have been designed with ALPs in mind. The exceptions are Big Macks or light-tech VOCAs (Voice Output Communication Aids) like GoTalks, which may have phrases rather than single words programmed into them.

For many years in the AAC world we have talked about the features of an AAC system which make it 'robust' (this being the chosen term for the 'gold standard'). The features of a robust AAC system have largely been agreed to be:

- Core-and-fringe vocabulary is available throughout the system. Core words are the everyday words which make up 80% of what we say. Core words include pronouns (I, you, he, she, it) and determiners (the, a), common verbs (go, eat, see, come), prepositions (to, up, on) and common adjectives or modifiers (big, more, gone). Fringe words are the words that are specific to a topic or situation. For example, food items, animals, clothes words.

- The system allows the person to express a range of communication intentions. For example, requesting, commenting, describing, asking and answering questions, giving an opinion.

- The system allows for language growth: it will allow the person to acquire more vocabulary and more complex grammar.

- The system has access to the alphabet so that the user can acquire literacy skills. They can learn to spell words, giving them access to an unlimited vocabulary.

- The system can be personalised for the user, and can be backed up to prevent possible loss of their personalisations. Personalisations include the choice of voice, the layout of cells on the package, the organisation of pages within the package, and the vocabulary and grammar choices.

What is the gold standard for GLP AAC?

This needs to be developed over the next few years, as we learn from GLPs about the features of an AAC system that are most important to them. This is likely to include:

- The ability to programme the AAC user's personal language gestalts in the AAC system. If the user is non-speaking, they may be indicating to us what their personal gestalts are through the movie clips that they rewind and rewatch, the songs that they love, and the phrases that they most respond to and want us to repeat for them.

- If the AAC user previously used spoken echolalia but then became minimally or non-speaking, we can use their previous scripts and programme these into the AAC system. If family have video of the child when they were younger, they may be able to recall previous language gestalts.

- If the AAC user has unreliable speech, that is that they do use speech sometimes, when they are well-regulated and rested, but sometimes their speech is difficult to access, then we will need to include their personal gestalts that they can sometimes say on their AAC system. They might choose to record these using message-banking. Therefore the AAC system needs to have the capacity to record original sound source.

- The AAC system will also offer access to any media clips that the AAC user derives gestalts from. This may be their favourite YouTube videos or music files. We will not 'lock down' their VOCA so that they can only access the AAC app.

- The vocabulary package that they are using will have the capacity to include phrases and longer chunks of language, alongside single words. These phrases might be organised by communication intention, e.g. 'expressing ideas', 'shared joy', 'describing', 'protesting', or they may be in the relevant topic page, so that the 'food' page has both single words for food items, and some phrases associated with eating and talking about food.

- The vocabulary package will have the capacity to support all of the stages of NLA. There will be stage 1 language gestalts. On the same page or a linked page, there will be the capacity to break down and mix-and-match these gestalts into mitigated gestalts. There will be referential words for stage 3, and capacity to combine core words with referential words to create stage 4–6 language.

- Most established AAC vocabulary packages already support stage 3 and 4 language. They have access to fringe words (stage 3 referential words) and core words (stage 4 and beyond).

- We do not want to completely reject existing robust AAC systems, because we want the AAC user to be able to go through stage 3 and stage 4 language using these packages. We will respect the way that the vocabulary package is organised, but we will add stage 1 and stage 2 language to existing pages, or an area of 'my phrases'.

- It is entirely possible that a child will be in stage 3 or beyond by the time they get an AAC system. Some children have managed to move through stage 1 and 2 language silently in their heads. By tracking their use of the AAC system using language samples, we can work out which stage they are 'living in' and support their AAC language accordingly.

- The option to add whole phrases into one button-press. Whole phrases from one button-press sound better. Try it out. Try formulating a message on a voice-output AAC system first by building word + word + word combinations. Try something like 'I did it!' Now try programming one cell with this whole phrase. Which one sounded more fun, natural and engaging? Unless technology has moved on since the writing of this book, I will bet that the whole-phrase-in-one-button option sounded more natural. A child in the first stages of their AAC journey is more likely to find AAC voice engaging and appealing if it sounds natural.

- The AAC system can be used flexibly to incorporate the other modes of communication that are important to the AAC user. If they like to arrange objects or capture images, we can experiment with incorporating this into the AAC system using visual scene displays. The AAC user might like having a writing or a drawing pad incorporated into their AAC. Clocks, timers, calendars and calculators are other options which may be desirable. These are all features that currently exist within robust AAC options.

Modelling AAC language

Just like we have to use spoken language in order for a child to absorb and process this, we have to use AAC language in order for a child to absorb and process this. The child will select the language that they take up. Some of it will stick, some of it won't. We want the language on the AAC system to be interesting and appealing, and we may experiment with child's preference for recorded sound from the original sound source, recorded speech with rich intonation, or using the digitised speech of the AAC software. The latter is much easier and less labour-intensive for programming, but initially, a child may engage better with recorded speech.

We will think about the communication intentions that a child is wanting to convey. 'Shared joy' or 'expressing ideas' are often a good place to start. We might choose a couple of phrases to model in an activity that the child really enjoys. For example, if they are loving our blowing up a balloon and letting it go, we can say 'I love it!' and 'that was fun!' using the AAC system. We will still use other spontaneous spoken language alongside our AAC language: we are modelling multi-modal communication.

For another child, we might start with a marble run, and model 'let's do it again!' and 'we need more'. For yet another child, we might start with their media gestalts whilst we watch some YouTube clips with them.

We model without expectation. We are not requiring the child to do anything in response. Just like with GLP spoken modelling, there is no 'eliciting' of language. There is no prompting, filling in the gap or offering fixed choices. If the child uses their AAC, they do it in their own time.

Engagement can take time

Initially a child may not look at their AAC. They need to check it out first. They may be doing this using their peripheral vision. They may just be listening, since we know that the auditory channel can be strong for GLPs.

We trust that the child has the capacity to take in this new modality for communication. We trust that they need to see what it might do for them before they take the plunge and use it.

AAC babble is valid!

Most children will initially 'babble' on their voice-output AAC. Having voice output is powerful! For the first time they can play with sounds. They may repeat-press one cell so that it repeats nonsense syllables over and over again. They may have a favourite phrase that they repeat over and over. They may systematically listen to each message in turn. They may run their whole hand across the screen with random selections. All of these are valid explorations of this new mode of communication, and we should delight in it, alongside the child.

Stimming with the device

Often adults will worry that the child is 'stimming' with the device, or even becoming dysregulated with excitement. Stimming is a valid and joyful self-expression. Consider whether it is the child who is dysregulated or the adults around the child. They are not used to the child being noisy. There may also be a cultural bias against digitised speech. If the child is very clearly becoming excited to the point of dysregulated, consider what other sensory supports might be put in place when they are exploring their voice. See Chapter 10 for 'calming activities'.

They will surprise us

We may notice a slight increase in the child glancing at the AAC. We may not. The first meaningful press of a button often takes us by surprise, just like a child's first mouth-word or phrase often takes us by surprise. We have a tendency to doubt the evidence in front of us when this happens. For some reason we often wonder if it was an accident, or a random press. The second time it happens there is no doubt. We will respond to this communication, just as we would if a child had used speech.

A new AAC user is not necessarily starting from stage 1

We know that non-speaking or minimally speaking children have language in their head that they cannot express with spoken words. When we provide AAC for the first time, we don't know where their language acquisition has led them so far. They might have a wealth of internal language gestalts. They might already be mitigating these. They might even have isolated words and be moving into pre-sentence and sentence grammar. By introducing a gold-standard AAC system we are offering access to language at various stages. Only by modelling and then observing (taking regular language samples) will we know what stage of language acquisition they are operating in. I have worked with many children who were able to create novel phrases from very early on in their AAC adventures.

Explore and integrate text-to-speech from the start

We always choose an AAC solution that includes access to the alphabet. On a paper-based AAC system, this will be an alphabet chart. On an app this will be an onscreen keyboard. My default layout is a QWERTY keyboard layout, as this will be replicated across the other apps and computer programmes the child uses.

Many apps also offer the option of a phonetic keyboard (that sounds out as the child types). We can remove the letter sounds once a child is getting proficient at typing. There is usually an option of including a bar of 'predictions' as the child is typing. Some children use these predictions to help them spell the whole word out, and this reinforces their literacy. They can also see the relationship between similarly spelled words, and different grammatical forms of certain words, e.g. 'walk', 'walks', 'walked', 'walking'.

As soon as a child shows interest in typing, we should go with this. We can model how to spell their name, the names of their family, pets, their favourite tv shows and so on. When we can't find a word on their symbol package, we should type it out, so that the child can see the value of the keyboard.

Often GLPs will enjoy us typing out their language gestalts, and perhaps some potential mitigations. If they are at stage 3 in their language, we can play games of referential naming using the keyboard. We can offer short phrases and sentences, showing stage 4 possibilities. We can show how we build phrases word by word. We can show grammatical constructions like verb endings, different pronouns, question forms and so on.

Ultimately, typing is a much quicker AAC option than navigating between pages and pages of symbols. It gives access to unlimited language and learning. See the second case study at the end of the chapter to see how text-to-speech AAC might unfold.

Paper-based AAC

Whilst an AAC app on an iPad is a brilliant way to introduce a child to AAC and voice output, there will also be times when they need paper-based AAC, because the iPad has run out of charge or cannot be used in a messy or wet environment.

Paper-based AAC has an obvious disadvantage, in that there is no voice output. There is a less obvious cause-and-effect relationship between what the child touches and other people noticing. However if it were a choice between paper-based AAC and no AAC, I know which I would prefer.

We do not want to provide paper-based AAC that has been designed for ALPs. Therefore core boards and 'core-and-fringe' communication books that consist of single words that can be combined to make phrases, are not going to be the best for a child who needs stage 1 or stage 2 language. Instead, we want the paper-based AAC to include potential stage 1 phrases, and the capacity to develop through stage 2 mitigations.

The great advantage that I find with paper-based AAC for stage 1 and 2 GLPs is that it is much less bulky than an ALP 'core-and-fringe' communication book. It is quicker to make and easy to make multiples for different settings.

Ideally the paper-based AAC will either replicate or closely resemble any high-tech AAC on an iPad. Many AAC apps allow us to simply print out pages of the app. If we don't want a bulky communication book, then I would suggest prioritising the home page, personal gestalts, phrases to cover the main functions of language and an alphabet chart.

AAC apps

All of the big AAC suppliers, Smartbox, TobiiDynavox, Liberator and AssistiveWare, offer robust AAC apps. AAC apps evolve, and what proves popular in one app generally makes it across into all the other apps. At the time of writing the following apps are regularly used with GLPs: Voco Chat and Super Core 50 (Grid for iPad), TD Snap (Tobii Dynavox), LAMP Words for Life (Liberator), Proloquo and Proloquo2Go (AssistiveWare).

At the time of writing all of the well-known apps have the capacity to add phrases into dedicated pages for 'My phrases' or into existing pages organised into topics. We want to respect the integrity of these well-designed apps, and so we won't make changes to the layout of the home page or the basic categories or topic pages. Instead we will add phrases to existing pages, or create an area for 'my phrases' and organise these by communication intention. Very likely we will use a combination of these strategies!

Some AAC apps have the capacity to add video clips directly into the vocabulary package or to toggle easily to YouTube. Many have the capacity to record original audio through message-banking. All the major apps have the capacity to personalise the package to include existing and potential language gestalts. Some have more room than others to be able to add mix-and-match stage 2 phrases into existing pages.

Text-to-speech AAC apps

Most children begin with a symbolised package, but then progress to a text-to-speech AAC package. This is the ultimate aim: that literacy will develop, giving the AAC user access to unlimited language. All AAC apps should include an onscreen keyboard, ideally with word or even phrase prediction. Often children will reach a point where they are preferring to type, and then we can think about moving them on to a text-to-speech app. At the time of writing, good options are Proloquo4Text (AssistiveWare), Predictable (Therapy box) and Fast Talker (Grid for iPad). See also the next chapter on 'GLP and literacy'.

Recognising language gestalts when a child is non-speaking

We want to use a child's personal language gestalts in their AAC. A speaking child will be reproducing gestalts by attempting to say them, but how do we recognise a non-speaking child's gestalts? We might see that they:

- Still their body and move in close to a particular line of a song, story or video clip.

- Show excitement in their body, by bouncing or rocking.

- Widen their eyes, or become more animated in their face.

- Look at us.

- Change their breathing pattern: it might pause or speed up, or there might be a gasp of excitement.

- Reach for us and show us in some way, by pointing or looking or taking our hand to the book or tablet.

- Vocalise in some way: a squeal or a yell, or something more subtle. They may mouth the words, or look like they are trying to.

- Engage with the gestalt over and over again: replaying the part in a video clip or acting out the part of a story or event.

- Show great excitement when we programme these soundtracks into their AAC, either using a recording of the original sound source, or matching our intonation pattern to the original as closely as possible.

How to organise a child's language gestalts

When we are adding a child's personal gestalt, we will think about their communication intention. GLPs are not literal at stage 1, so we would not store it according to the literal meaning of the words. We will think about the intended meaning or language function of the phrase.

If a child has a gestalt 'there's more beyond the reef', a quote from Moanna, and they seem to use it to give reassurance to themselves, then this can be added into a page for 'self-advocacy' or 'self-talk'. If they use the phrase 'like the break of dawn' when they are happy, we will add this to their 'shared joy' page.

Paper-based stage 1: what might it look like?

Stage 1 paper-based GLP-friendly AAC will likely be organised into communication intentions. Each page will have phrases to model for different communication intentions: expressing ideas, expressing shared joy, describing, protesting, managing transitions, expressing sensory needs and self-advocacy. The child's personal gestalts will be organised into these communication intentions as much as possible. If we are not yet sure of the intended meaning, they may be on a separate page.

It can be helpful to colour-code the tables in a book, so that each page is associated with a different colour. This doesn't mean anything linguistically, but makes each page memorable and distinct.

In Figure 12.1 is a sample page of a stage 1 GLP-friendly communication book. This page offers phrases themed around the communication intention of 'expressing ideas'.

You can find the template for the complete book by visiting the website at the beginning of this book (along with other supplementary handouts). You can also see the template on my Instagram page, ali_battye_speech.

Ideally we will replicate the paper-based AAC layout in a 'my phrases' page in a high-tech AAC app. So from the home page there will be a jump to 'my phrases' and this can then be organised into the communication intentions, with a page of phrases for each function.

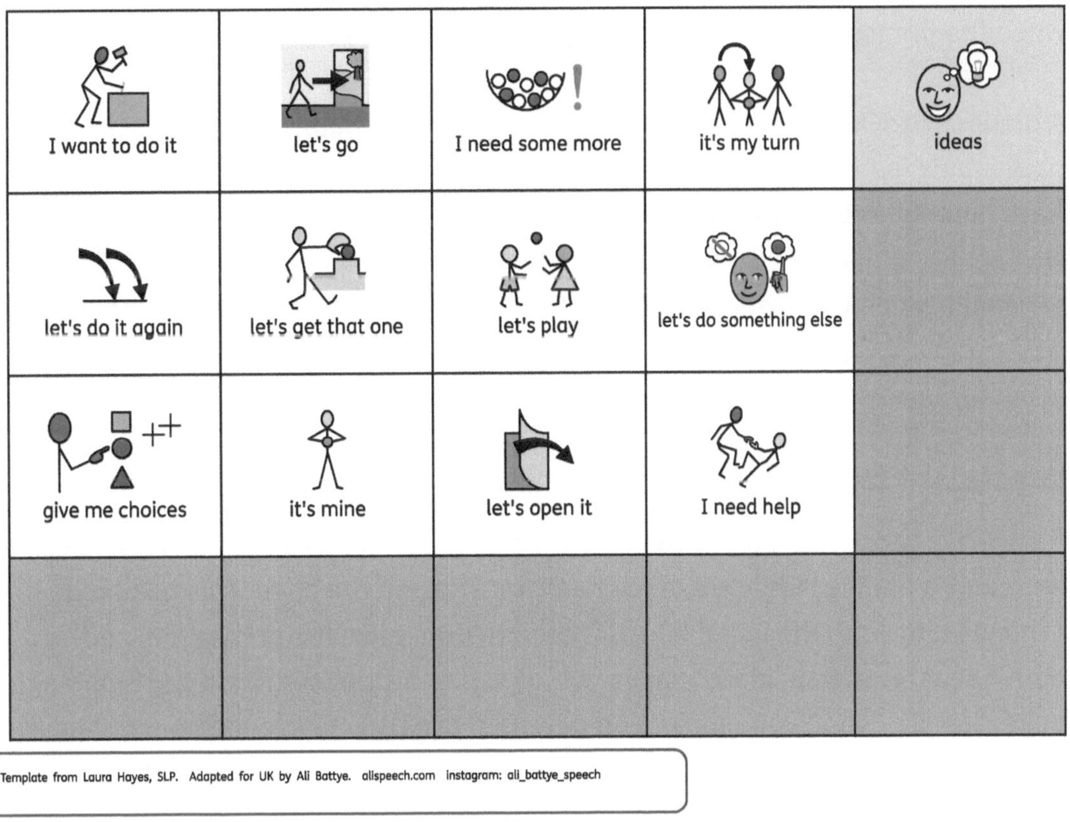

I want to do it	let's go	I need some more	it's my turn	ideas
let's do it again	let's get that one	let's play	let's do something else	
give me choices	it's mine	let's open it	I need help	

Template from Laura Hayes, SLP. Adapted for UK by Ali Battye. alispeech.com instagram: ali_battye_speech

Figure 12.1 GLP-friendly communication book 'ideas' page

©Widgit Symbols 2002–2024

Some phrases may sit within the main communication app. For example, a child's gestalt 'yummy scrummy for my tummy', will sit within the food page. We will make these case-by-case decisions for each child, because each child's stage 1 language is different.

Stage 1 language may include video clips and recorded speech. For paper-based AAC, we might screenshot the video clip so that there is an image to accompany the child's gestalt.

To symbolise or not?

You will notice that the example pages have been symbolised. But we do not want to over-symbolise. For stage 1 language, we will find a symbol that expresses the 'overall feeling' of the phrase. We certainly would not want a 'word for word' symbol translation, because a stage 1 GLP does not have that 'word for word' literal understanding. They are understanding the whole of it, and the whole is more than the sum of its parts.

For the child's naturally acquired gestalts, I do not think a symbol could capture the 'whole of it'. If the gestalt is from a media clip, we could screenshot the moment when the phrase is spoken and have this alongside the text.

A distinctive symbol or screenshot for a message may help with visual scanning, particularly for the supporting adults, but don't assume that symbols or pictures have inherent meaning for the GLP.

We could experiment with text-only AAC. For hyperlexic children, this is probably the best option. We can colour-code pages to make each page visually distinctive. This is not for linguistic reasons, but to help with navigation.

Consistent layout for motor planning

If messages are duplicated across multiple pages of the AAC system, it is helpful for motor planning if they are in the same location on the page. This is difficult to achieve, but worth the initial effort. Therefore if we have the phrase 'let's go!' in both 'ideas' and 'transitions' pages, we want it to occupy the same position on the page. The child (and communication partners) can use muscle memory to find the same message, rather than having to actively scan a whole page of phrases.

Stage 1 AAC gestalts are sometimes multiple cell presses

I have noticed a tendency in my AAC-using GLPs that they will be brilliant at memorising and using navigational pathways, and will initially reproduce the same sequence of button-presses to make the same message over and over.

For example, Ella, who is featured in the case study at the end of this chapter, loves to combine two phrases in her 'shared joy' page. She said 'I like it' + 'I love you' as her original stage 1 gestalt. She used these two button presses together consistently for about two months. She then started to 'mix-and-match' them with other phrases on this page, e.g. 'I like it' + 'we're having fun', or 'it's my favourite' + 'I love you'. She also sometimes used just one of these phrases: another form of mitigation.

Adapting an ALP package for a GLP: planning for stage 2

We are all experimenting at this point in time, and so I want to share some other ways that I have been adapting AAC packages for GLPs. In Figures 12.2 and 12.3 are two screenshots from the 'Grid for iPad' package, Voco Chat. The first screenshot is

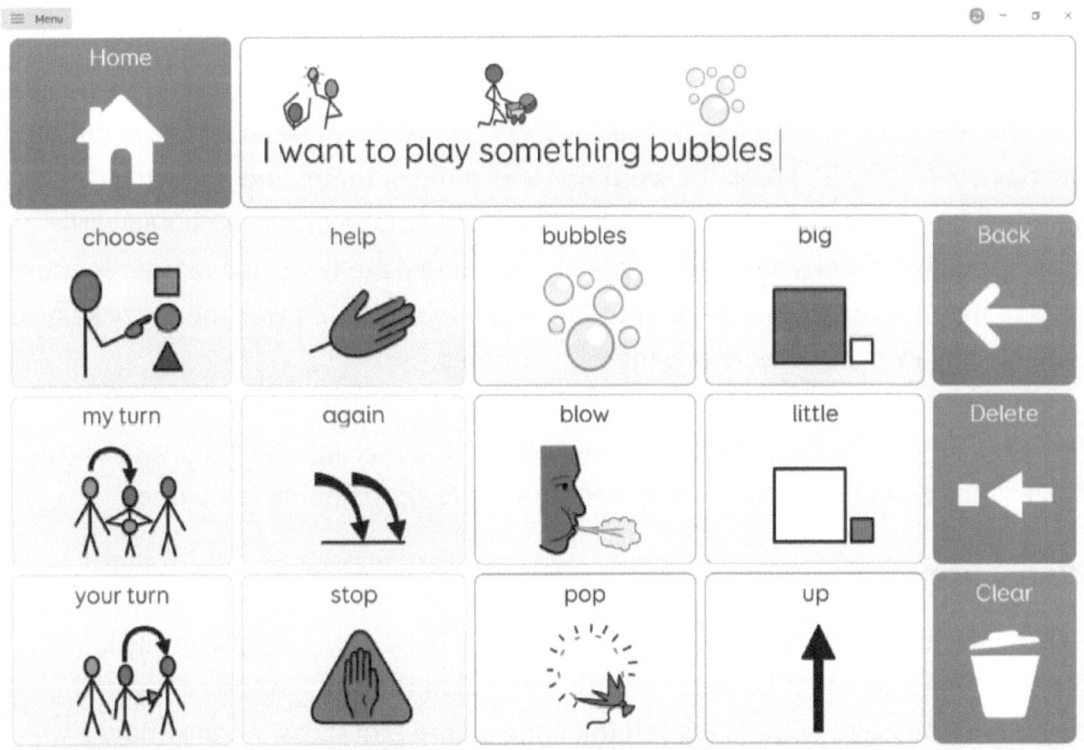

Figure 12.2 Voco Chat 'bubbles' page: the original ALP version

©Widgit Symbols 2002–2024

Reproduced with permission from Smartbox

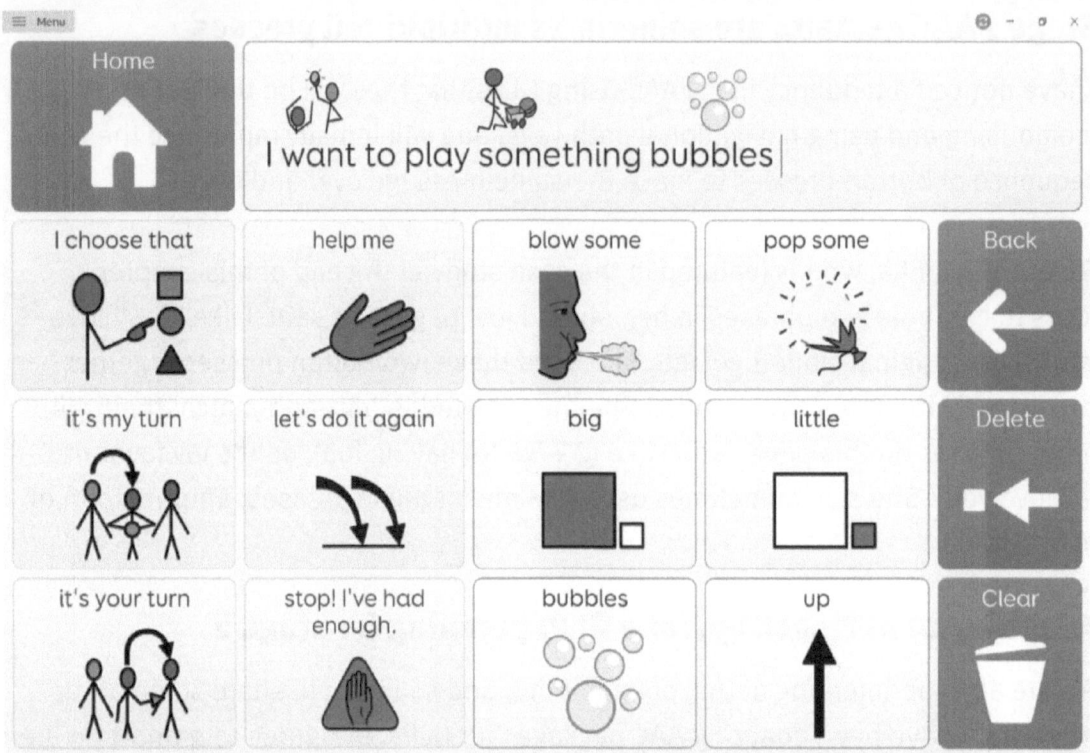

Figure 12.3 Voco Chat 'bubbles' page: the edited GLP-friendly version

©Widgit Symbols 2002–2024

Reproduced with permission from Smartbox

how the ALP original page looks. The second screenshot shows how I have edited the page to 'GLPify it'. I took the word that was already there, and if it worked, I made it into a short phrase that could either stand alone or be combined with other language chunks or single words on the same page (I've also rearranged some cells to help language flow better, but this is not essential). It was then very easy to use this page whilst we were playing with bubbles.

Not all GLPs will need these edits. If they are moving through the stages and have stage 3 and 4 language, they will benefit from core words being left alone.

Visual scenes

Another layout option is to have 'visual scenes' (Figure 12.4). This typically takes the form of a photo that is personally meaningful to the child at the centre of the page, with message buttons around the edge or into 'hotspots' on the image, programmed with meaningful phrases to accompany the image.

This is a good option for valuing a child's favourite visual media or their own creations. For example, if they love arranging treasured objects, or looking at

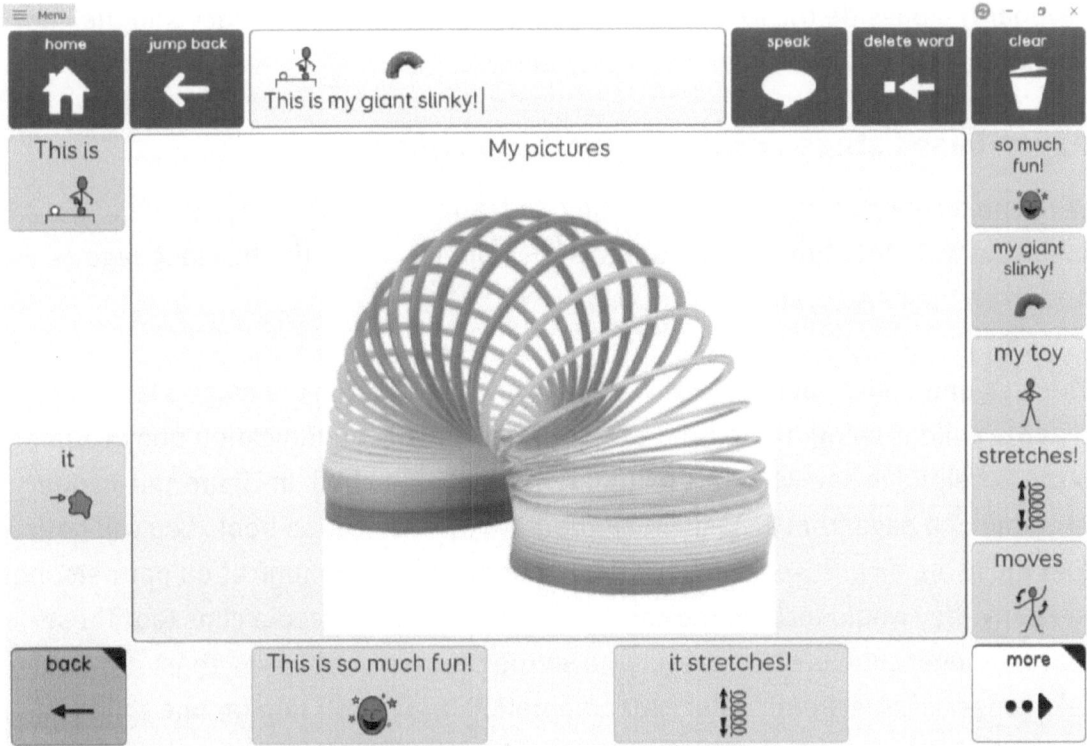

Figure 12.4 Visual scene display

©Widgit Symbols 2002–2024

Reproduced with permission from Smartbox

scenes from unusual angles, we might photograph this, and then programme some phrases around it. For example, 'This is so much fun!', 'it stretches!' It is also possible (and recommended) to include some options for mitigations, e.g. 'This is' + 'so much fun!' 'my giant slinky!' or 'my toy'; 'it' + 'stretches' or 'moves'.

Show the child the 'delete' and 'backspace' functions

Some children will spontaneously work out that they can delete a word or a language chunk from a longer phrase. This allows them to mitigate. They can reduce down a longer chunk of language, and they can 'mix-and-match' from there. As they get to know their AAC package and their navigation between pages increases, the possibilities for mitigation take off. A well-designed AAC package will have useful links between pages of vocabulary, and will include well-placed links to the onscreen keyboard.

The importance of an onscreen keyboard

There is infinite possibility for mitigation when we model typing as an option. We are always offering and modelling text-to-speech AAC (using the onscreen keyboard) alongside the symbolised AAC. Our ultimate aim is literacy and the unlimited access to language that typing allows.

Paper-based stage 2: what might it look like?

With spoken language, we wait for a child to lead us into their stage 2 language. It is the same with AAC, but we will want to anticipate this and offer this language as an option on their AAC system.

The 'mix-and-match' options that we offer will depend upon the stage 1 language that the child is using. There is no prescribed stage 2 communication book content, but it is helpful to see what this might look like for one child. In Figure 12.5 is one example of a page from a stage 2 GLP-friendly communication book. You will notice that these are all phrases that have been modelled by communication partners, but in reality they would include the child's own gestalts from media clips too. These may be longer chunks of language, and so the process of trimming them down may take longer. This is a process of experimentation, and a solution for one child will not be the same as the solution for another. As with all AAC, there is a big element of trial and error.

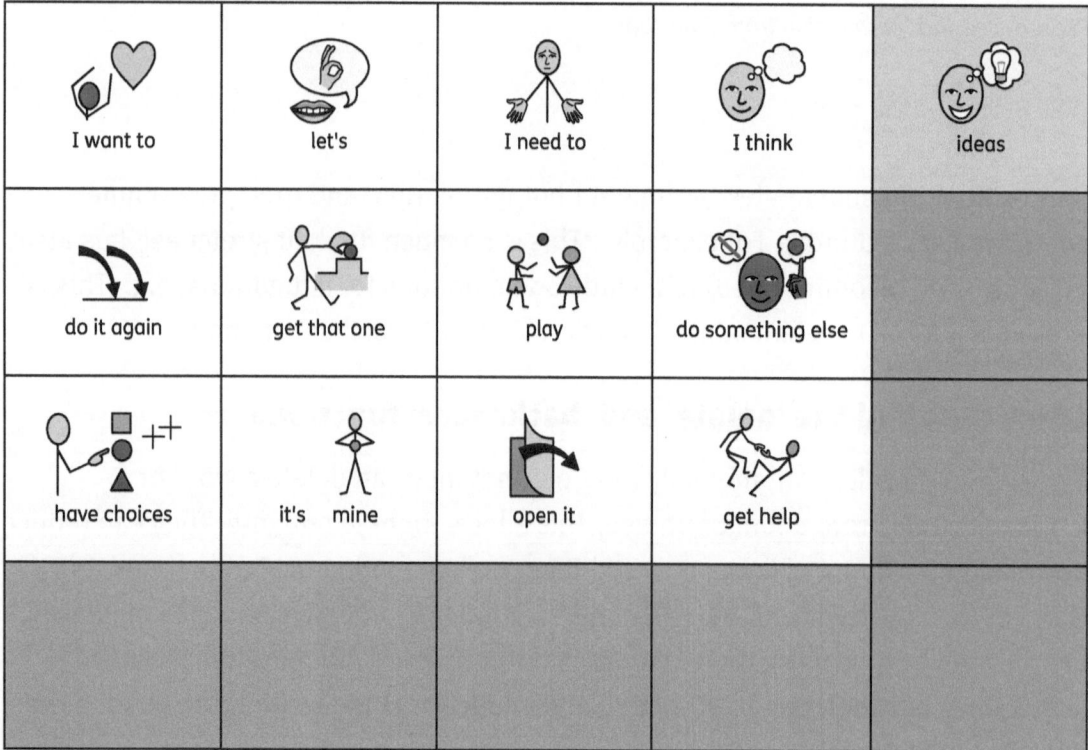

Figure 12.5 GLP-friendly communication book 'ideas' page with stage 2 mitigations

©Widgit Symbols 2002–2024

Stage 1 and stage 2 language might share the same page

This is where a communication app with lots of space on a page is helpful. If there is space, we might have stage 2 language on the same page as stage 1 language. In the 'shared joy' page, we might have stage 1 gestalt 'it's a beautiful day!' Alongside this we could create buttons with 'it's', 'a beautiful day', 'so much fun' and 'my favourite'. Be as creative as possible with the options in stage 2, thinking about the child's interests, sensory, movement and play preferences. Their personal stage 1 language will provide inspiration.

'Jumps' to other pages

If we feel that stage 3 is just around the corner, we will want to create a 'jump' button which leads to stage 3 language. This might be the 'topics' page or the 'home' page. The jump button could equally lead to the onscreen keyboard, allowing us to model the spellings for referential words that the child is pointing to.

The child will always need access to their stage 1 and 2 language, so we won't delete this once they make the leap into stage 3 and 4 language. These express their personality and their language heritage.

Mitigating media gestalts

If a child has media gestalts programmed into their AAC app, we will want to retain the original sound source recording, and we may also offer trimmed down versions, or versions where the audio is the device's digitised speech. This variation is a potential mitigation.

We can monitor a child's readiness for this: I have worked with a child who initially rejected any form of mitigation, but then became happy to for me to trim these down using my voice instead of the original sound source recording: a sign of entering stage 2. This was accompanied by interest in other phrases on the AAC system that did not originate from media gestalts. There was a general readiness for greater variety in stage 1, alongside early mitigation.

Stage 3 and beyond

Since apps have generally been designed with ALPs in mind, they are naturally suited to stage 3 referential language, with folders full of nouns, attributes and locations. A robust AAC system will have access to 'core-and-fringe' vocabulary, which leads us nicely into stage 4. If you look at the screen shot in Figure 12.6, you can see how stage 4 language can be generated from the home page of a package.

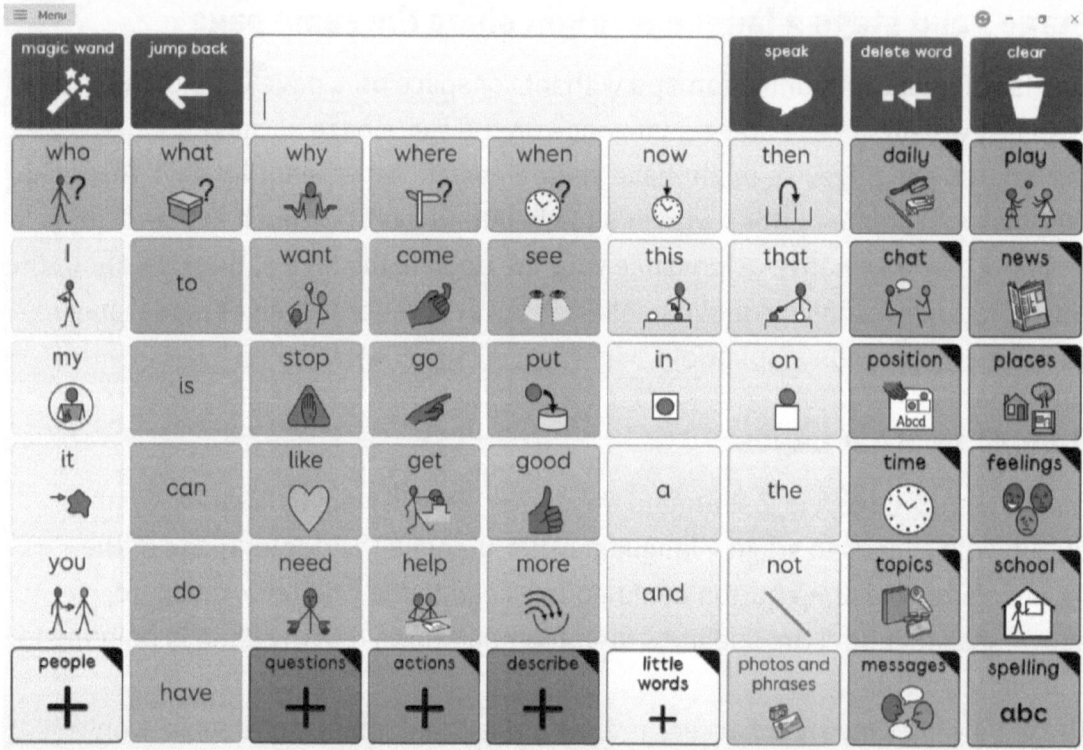

Figure 12.6 Super Core 50 home page

©Widgit Symbols 2002–2024

Reproduced with permission from Smartbox

Other packages have core words arranged differently, but all robust AAC vocabulary packages have core words that are easily accessible, either on the home page or within other pages, with consistent locations for motor planning where possible. Another alternative is that we show the child how to type these words, as part of their literacy learning (see Chapter 13 for more on literacy).

'Core-and-fringe' language allows for stage 3 and 4 development

Adult AAC users have told us that AAC helped them to segment the sound-stream into separate words. A traditional 'core-and-fringe' robust AAC package shows a child visually how a phrase is made up of a word + a word + a word. And so AAC can help a child make a leap into stage 3 referential language, and into stage 4 word + word + word constructions.

Allowing a child to simply explore their robust AAC system, which not only has stage 1 gestalts and stage 2 mitigations, but also has stage 3 and 4 'core-and-fringe' words will support this natural process. From time to time we can model single words or word + word combinations. We never know when a child is ready to move into the next stage. AAC language development often takes us by surprise because so much of the language acquisition is happening in a child's head.

Part-time AAC

Many autistic adults use AAC part time when they are tired, ill or dysregulated. Therefore we want to offer AAC as an option even if an autistic person is speaking using mouth-words for much of the time. If families notice that there are times when the child cannot seem to access their speech, then we will need to consider AAC. We don't know the benefit they will get until we try it.

Visual supports

Do GLPs need visual supports? It depends.

A lot depends upon the intention. If the visual support is to give the child structure and reassurance and help them understand how long an activity will go on for; if it is to prepare them for a new experience or a change in the usual routine; if they seem to benefit from this visual support, then we can offer visual supports such as a visual timetable, a social story, a visual timer, a clock or a calendar.

If the intention of a visual support is to urge compliance or defer their access to sensory regulation, then this is not acceptable. For example, a 'now-and-next' board where they finish their spellings and then get a fidget toy. Sensory and movement breaks and equipment should not be used as a reward but should be available to the child to help them attend and regulate throughout the day.

Summary of AAC supports

- Introduce a robust AAC system that is adapted for GLPs, taking into consideration their current gestalts and planning for future mitigations.

- Experiment with the sound source that they find most appealing, be it a recording from the original sound source, recording speech with rich intonation or using the digitised speech of the AAC system.

- Experiment with the visual appearance. Consider visual scene displays in order to value the visual media that the child is drawn to, or those they create themselves, e.g. photos, arrangements of objects.

- Incorporate the child's enthusiasms and favourite activities, and programme personalised language around these.

- Experiment with useful short phrases to express a range of communication intentions, e.g. sharing ideas, expressing shared joy, describing and so on.

- Provide useful short phrases which may be mix-and-matched for potential stage 2 mitigations.

- Introduce one or two pages of this AAC system in fun activities. Model phrases like 'I like it!', 'we did it', 'let's do it again', 'what's next?' to match the child's likely communication intention.

- Model without expectation: children need to see us using and valuing the AAC system first. They may not even look at it initially: this is fine.

- Continue to also use natural speech; we can use a rich mixture of spoken language modelling plus AAC language modelling.

- The first signs of engagement with AAC might be pressing all the buttons at once, repeat-pressing the same button, 'stimming' using the AAC. This is all fine. It shows engagement and interest.

- Consider the use of a paper-based AAC system which may replicate the key pages of the iPad-based AAC.

- Plan for stage 2 mitigations: think about using visual scene displays or programming both stage 1 and stage 2 language on the same page.

- Include an onscreen keyboard and alphabet chart so that the child has access to this. This is important for literacy acquisition and ultimately for limitless language use.

- Model navigation between pages of vocabulary, and model using the 'delete' and 'backspace' functions. Show how we can use the onscreen keyboard when we can't find the word or the language chunk that we need. This prepares a child to move beyond stage 1 language, through stage 2 mitigations, and into stages 3 and 4.

- Continue to respond to communication in all modalities: body posture, proximity, vocalisations, hand-leading, speech, AAC, what the child is showing us through their play, chosen media, movement and sensory activities.

- Allow for time to programme the robust AAC system for the child. Initial personalisation might take one to two hours, and then allow six to ten hours per year from there.

- Respect the integrity of the robust AAC system as you make tweaks for a GLP.

- It is not sufficient to put an AAC system in front of a child and expect them to use it. They need to see us using it and valuing it. AAC language acquisition can be a lengthy process, just like spoken language acquisition. Regular and long-term Speech and Language Therapy input is needed.

- A child needs to hear at least 200 models of AAC use per day. This is not as hard as it sounds, since in one interaction we may use ten phrases. That's 20 interactions of ten phrases, or any other distribution through the school day. AAC use is woven into the ordinary interactions that any child has at school, little and often.

Case study: Ella

Ella's mum, Louise, contacted me to discuss possible therapy for her daughter. Ella attended a local special school. She was 9 years old. She was described as 'non-speaking'. Ella had been accessing Intensive Interaction for several years. She had a core-and-fringe communication book, and she could use this to request favourite food items and toys. Ella's mum felt that Ella wanted to speak, but that her development had stalled. Louise sent me some videos of Ella vocalising: she was watching her mum talk and she was trying to copy mouth shapes, but she was not achieving voice at the same time.

Ella's mum told me that Ella loves small items, particularly those that are circular or disc-shaped, and also collecting pairs of objects, e.g. drumsticks.

These are my notes from our first session:

Ella attended for her first therapy session with Louise, her mum. Ella was initially hesitant, but on seeing toys she engaged immediately.

Ella loved the coloured marbles and cupcakes, spreading out the marbles, gathering them up and putting them in the cups. She also loved the chopsticks, and used these as drumsticks, playing the drums on boxes, pans, etc. She loved the piano too, listening intently and trying out high and low notes. She also liked the coloured lights and pretend food, especially the two lollipops and the ice-creams (Louise says she loves pairs of items).

Ella was very communicative, using her actions, face and vocalisations to make her message clear, e.g. 'this one's for you', 'I've got two of them'. There were periods where she was quiet, and periods where she vocalised with open vowel sounds, and the odd semivowel (w y). During one exchange, I shaped a vocalisation into 'oh yeah' and Ella carried on with this for five or six turns.

I modelled a few messages on the paper-based GLP communication book and on the iPad Voco Chat app. Ella was more interested in the book today, but this may have been because the whole experience was new and she was just settling in. Ella used her own core-and-fringe communication book spontaneously, pointing to items on her 'treats' page.

Ella was very comfortable exploring the space. She likes to crawl across the room, and under tables and chairs, and often had her head upside down (which is her instinct I guess for vestibular and proprioceptive input). She also plonked herself in my lap and enjoyed that proximity.

Although we are early on in our journey together, I feel that we can use movement and child-led play to:

- *Encourage and repeat back vocalisations, bringing in increased volume and variation of sounds.*

- *Assume that Ella is saying words: give her the benefit of the doubt, and copy it back as a word.*

- *Explore the use of the GLP communication book for phrases: maybe focus first on the pages for 'Shared Joy' and 'Regulation'.*

- *Explore the use of the GLP Voco Chat package on the iPad, using the same pages for 'Shared Joy' and 'Regulation'.*

- *We're not expecting Ella to use the communication book or iPad yet: just to experience adults around her using it to express her likely communication intentions.*

In the following session, Ella began to explore the iPad app. She pressed a few buttons repeatedly, enjoying the voice-output. Our therapy sessions had a rhythm that was set by Ella: she would have a burst of movement and being very vocal. I would assume that she was saying a phrase, and would copy that back for her. This appeared to delight Ella. Then Ella would be quiet and focused for a while, and we might model some phrases on her iPad which seemed to match her communication intention, e.g. 'look at that', and 'I like it'. When Ella needed to move, we modelled 'need to spin' and 'let's dance'.

By the third session, Louise reported that Ella had just said 'more' very clearly in the car. Other family members had noticed that Ella was communicating more. She was seeking people out, showing them items of interest and making sure that they were noticing what she was doing.

Ella vocalised something that sounded very much like 'look!' in this session. Later, when Louise modelled 'let's do it again', Ella very deliberately looked at the iPad and pressed 'let's play!'

In our fourth session, Ella pressed the button for 'let's go' and then pressed it a second time, and looked at us.

Louise expressed concern in the next session that Ella was not particularly looking at the iPad when family members were modelling its use. However we did notice her glancing very briefly at it, and in that session, Ella used her iPad to say, 'I want a cuddle'. She went to her mum to confirm that she very definitely wanted a cuddle. At the end of the session, Ella once again said 'let's go'.

Over the next few sessions, Ella added to her repertoire of AAC gestalts. She frequently said, 'let's do it again' and 'I want to do it' with toys like the balloon pump and bubbles. She had a few gestalts of two button presses for 'I like it' + 'I love you'. She regularly said, 'need to spin', 'let's dance' and 'I want a tickle'. She was regularly using messages across a number of communication intentions, including sharing ideas, shared joy, describing, transitions and regulation.

If Ella had made a mistake by pressing a button and realising it was not the message she had intended, she would find the right button and press it three or four times, whilst looking at us, to show us that this is what she had really meant to say. Ella was also sometimes pressing each button in turn on a given page of her iPad AAC, and listening to each message. She would then select the one that she wanted, e.g. 'I feel calm' and look at us to indicate that this was the one she wanted.

At the same time, Ella's vocalisations were becoming louder and more varied. She was producing vowel sounds with intonation contours, using consonants that we had not heard before and attempting more mouth-words.

We now had a good idea of which phrases or sequences of phrases were gestalts for Ella when using her AAC. There were possibly some examples of mitigations, where she had moved from always pressing the same two buttons in the same order, to just pressing one of them, and mix-and-matching the sequence with other buttons.

We started to use a few pages that had whole phrases, mix-and-match phrases and single words, including the 'bubbles' page shown earlier in this chapter. Ella enjoyed exploring these messages, as well as us modelling them to her.

We followed Ella's lead in our play-based sessions. Interestingly, her play choices widened. It was as if her whole world was opening up. If she was interested in pretend food, we took her to the food pages of her AAC. If she was interested in miniature animals, we took her to those pages. She often pressed each button in turn on a new page, as if she were learning or matching the words to her experience of the world. She showed a preference for some items on each page, perhaps liking the sound of the word, and also showing her interest in specific items. For example, she loved the word 'tomato', and clearly delighted in this word. She also showed us that she recognised a match between a word on her AAC and the item she was holding, saying 'turtle' and holding it up for us to see.

This was our cue to explore building 'word + word' combinations, using the core and fringe words on the AAC. Fortunately we had chosen a robust AAC app from the start, which allowed us to easily extend into this territory. We started to use words in the 'describing' pages, 'position' pages, 'actions' and 'quick words', which allowed us to model isolated words like 'more', 'big', 'here' and 'gone', and word + word combinations like 'ball again' and 'big bubble'.

Ella still had a lot of her AAC vocabulary package to explore, but already she was well on her way to being able to express a range of communication intentions. People were already viewing her differently, and, perhaps in response to this, Ella was holding her head up more, sharing her space with others, showing them what she was interested in and what she was doing, and regularly vocalising, attempting words or phrases, and using her iPad to express her thoughts and feelings.

Case study: Jenson

Jenson's dad Chris contacted me when he noticed one day that Jenson had come home from his school (a large specialist school for children with diverse learning needs) and had drawn a picture of a plate with food on it, and then he had written 'eat dinner'. Up until then, no one knew that Jenson could read, let alone write. Jenson was non-speaking, with diagnoses of autism and ADHD. He struggled with school, having moved class several times due to 'behaviour' and he was currently on a reduced timetable. Jenson's communication options at school were limited to PECS. His parents reported that he did not engage with PECS at home. They had lost count of the times they had retrieved it from the bin.

Because Chris had given me a hint that Jenson was able to read and write, or at least could write two words, I prepared for our session by getting out a whiteboard and pens, my iPad with a couple of different AAC apps, including Super Core, a symbol package with an onscreen keyboard, and various toys and books around his interests. I knew that Jenson loved dinosaurs and animals.

Jenson pushed the iPad away when I tried to show him the symbolised AAC app. However he loved the whiteboard and pens, and started drawing dinosaurs and animals, copying these from an Eric Carle Amazing Book of Animals. I used the onscreen keyboard of the AAC app to try to guess the animal Jenson was drawing. He glanced at what I was doing from the corner of his eye, and then smiled at my guesses. Jenson started to challenge me with ever more obscure animals, as I typed my guesses: 'flamingo . . . ostrich . . . vulture' and so on. Jenson found this hilarious and beat his fists on his chest in delight when I correctly guessed an animal.

Over the next week, Jenson's parents loaded a personalised version of the AAC app onto Jenson's iPad. When they returned the following week, Jenson's parents reported that he had been using the AAC app to talk about animals, using both the symbols and the onscreen keyboard. He was using the symbols, looking at the word there and then he went to the keyboard to type the word out. He had also produced further drawings, writing the label beneath the animal: 'chimpanzee', 'ferret' and 'musk ox'.

After just a week, Jenson's navigation was already impressive: when we looked at the Eric Carle book and Jenson typed 'kangaroo', I said 'it has a baby in its pouch'. Jenson promptly navigated to the 'animal babies' page in Super Core, and selected 'joey'.

In this session we used a reuseable sticker book and Jenson very thoughtfully placed animals in the correct habitats: rainforest, savannah, ocean and so on. I then typed the name of the animal and said a short phrase, e.g. 'Giraffe. Drinking water from the pool', 'Monkey. Swinging through the trees'. I didn't know what stage of NLA Jenson was in, so I was hedging my bets by modelling phrases alongside the single words that he was clearly interested in.

Jenson then sought out the Eric Carle book and used this to check my spellings! He chose animal stickers with longer names: 'orangutan', 'antelope' and 'wildebeest'. He found it funny when a spelling eluded me. I tried to explain my reasoning when I was struggling with a spelling, and drawing attention to words that were similar, e.g. 'orangutan' starts like 'orange'. The predictions above the keyboard encouraged this conversation.

Jenson then put the wildebeest sticker next to the musk ox picture in the Eric Carle book, showing that they were similar. I wondered if he was at least in stage 3 of NLA: he was showing an interest in matching and comparing two items, as well as pointing and showing.

Over the next week, Jenson's parents reported that Jenson was typing out animal names. Within the session he showed that he understood the correspondence between uppercase and lowercase letters, copy-typing the uppercase animal names from the Eric Carle book into his lowercase onscreen keyboard. The only letters he sometimes confused were uppercase 'I' with lowercase 'l'.

I continued to model phrases with Jenson. I created some visual scenes of his favourite animals from the Eric Carle book, for example the chimpanzees, and then some potential stage 1 and stage 2 options around the edges of the main image. Jenson beat his chest in delight when I showed him these. He pressed 'they're picking fleas' a few times. These new visual scenes were as yet on my iPad and not Jenson's iPad. I emailed the update to his mum that evening, and she told me that Jenson had stood over her until she successfully uploaded these onto his iPad!

I had shown Jenson how to add an '-s' ending onto his animal words, and when Jenson came for his next therapy session his parents said that he had been doing this a lot, and noticing that the corresponding symbol in the message window then changed to two animals. Again, this suggested to me that he had gone beyond stages 1 and 2 in his language development: he was interested in modulation of meaning through grammar.

Jenson spent this session typing animals with multi-part names, like 'rocky mountain goat', 'snow leopard', 'water buffalo' and 'red wolf'. I wondered if he was naturally exploring stage 3 language, with nouns and attributes. Jenson was showing me that he knew what he needed to do next: I just had to stay present to what he was showing me. Nevertheless, I did add a few more visual scenes around these new animals: I wanted to ensure that I was offering plenty of variety in stages 1 and 2.

At the end of this session, Jenson took up the whiteboard and returned to challenging me with drawing animals whilst I tried to guess what they were. I was struggling with an animal, and so Jenson typed 'pon . . .' on his iPad and then got stuck. His parents also tried to guess, but we were at a loss. Later that day, Jenson's mum sent me a video of Jenson typing 'pomeranian' twice on his iPad, and then laughing and beating his chest.

Jenson's typing speed was noticeably increasing, and he was holding whole words in his head now, without always needing to copy-type.

In our next session, Jenson found a very old app on my iPad: 'Pogg'. In this app we can either choose from a picture display or type an action word that we want Pogg, a green alien, to carry out. Pogg has endearingly large eyes and buck teeth, and a very funny range of facial expressions, and often has unfortunate accidents whilst carrying out these actions. I showed Jenson how he could type a word like 'hop' or 'jump' or 'eat', and Pogg would do this. Jenson up until this point had only been typing nouns (mainly animals, but also words like 'rainforest', 'ocean' and 'snow') and attributes (often colours). He continued to type nouns and attributes, and was amused when Pogg scratched his head in confusion.

I showed Jenson the 'actions' words on his AAC app, and I showed him how he could copy-type these too. He pushed my hand away, as he often did when I showed him something new, but, as had also happened many times before, the next week, he did this himself. Now he was typing 'throw', 'climb' and 'catch' alongside other types of words into the app. I showed him the function in Super Core where we can add different verb tenses to change 'jump' into 'jumps', 'jumping' or 'jumped'. Jenson glanced, like he so often did, and I suspected that the following week he would be using this function.

Jenson's parents told me that his interests were expanding: he was exploring YouTube videos about the solar system and atomic structure!

At this point, I liaised with Jenson's class teacher, who could instantly identify how she might be able to model language around his regulation needs in class. We talked about his literacy, and how text-to-speech AAC was supporting this. She was keen to start spending some one-to-one time with Jenson, following the same principles of child-led engagement using Jenson's interests.

I had only been working with Jenson for six sessions, but he had already shown me that he was open to modelling of stage 1 and 2 language via visual scenes, and that he was using referential stage 3 language via symbols and typing. He was showing me that he was interested in grammar. I was confident that we were about to start exploring stage 4 language. My job was to continue to allow Jenson to lead, to offer activities around his interests and to know that he would show me what he needed next.

Notes

1 Millar, D. C., Light, J. C. & Schlosser, R. W. (2006, April) 'The impact of augmentative and alternative communication intervention on the speech production of individuals with developmental disabilities: A research review' *Journal of Speech Language and Hearing Research* 49(2), 248–264.
2 Brignell, A., Chenausky, K. V., Song, H., Zhu, J., Suo, C. & Morgan, A. T. (2018, November 5) 'Communication interventions for autism spectrum disorder in minimally verbal children' *Cochrane Database of Systematic Review* 11.

Chapter 13

GLP and literacy

'I've never met an autistic child who doesn't love learning'.

Source unknown

In this chapter we will begin with hyperlexia, and then move on to literacy supports for all GLPs. As the quotation at the start of this chapter implies, all children have a right to literacy instruction. Our current education system prioritises phonics as the entry point into literacy, and we will learn in this chapter that this does not always align with a GLP's natural entry point into literacy. This chapter aims to provide options for these children. I hope that it may be useful for parents, Speech and Language Therapists and teaching staff.

Just as we presume communicative competence, we presume the potential to acquire literacy. We know that autistic children are often strong visual processors. We know that GLPs learn in 'wholes' first. This chapter is all about applying this knowledge to literacy acquisition.

Hyperlexia and GLP

More research is needed, but there seems to be a higher incidence of hyperlexia in GLPs than ALPs. Hyperlexia is the ability to read with minimal instruction having been provided, and the ability to read well in advance of similar aged peers.

Signs that a GLP may also be hyperlexic

- They spontaneously read words or phrases, without having been taught them.
- They have a strong interest in logos, letters and print from an early age.
- They like having closed captions or subtitles on when watching tv.
- They use alphabet magnets or blocks to spell out words they've only ever seen in print.
- They can correctly point to words that you ask them to.
- They quickly work out passwords and parental controls on technology!
- They notice if we don't read all the words in a story book.

DOI: 10.4324/9781032717029-13

Supports for a hyperlexic GLP

If a child is naturally drawn to written text, we honour this. We will support them in all the ways we would for a non-hyperlexic child (establishing trust and connection, being child-led and play-based in our approach, acknowledging their natural language). We just prioritise the modality of written text, in addition to our spoken language modelling.

- In addition to repeating back their words and phrases using speech, we also write them on a whiteboard or paper or type them into an AAC app.

- We provide access to magnetic letters and word tiles, and allow them to recreate words or phrases that they may have seen in the environment.

- We join them in their passion for the alphabet or logos, or written text in the environment.

- We show them how their spoken language can be translated into written text.

- At stage 1 we write down their gestalts. We might create a communication book made up of their gestalts, represented in text, and arranged by communication intention.

- At stage 2 we write down their mitigations. We might model other options for mitigation, mix-and-matching, or showing frame-and-slot constructions.

- At stage 3 we write down their single words and their word + word combinations. We can also match written words to pictures, label objects in the environment with written text on cards, or spell the words with magnetic letters.

- At stage 4 and beyond we write down their self-generated sentences.

- We provide them with written materials to support their learning, taking their enthusiasms as our starting point. Books might include picture dictionaries, non-fiction texts, story books, magazines, written instructions, recipes and so on.

- We explore making books together: photo books of days out or scrapbooks of favourite pictures, with some short captions that are personalised for the child.

- We turn on subtitles or closed captions when we are watching tv or accessing YouTube.

- We provide access to an onscreen keyboard on an iPad, and we show them how we can search subjects of interest (making use of appropriate parental controls for content).

- We provide a text-to-speech AAC app if the child has unreliable or unclear speech.

- We provide access to a paper-based alphabet chart if the child cannot yet use handwriting to create written text.

Literacy supports for GLPs

Hyperlexic children need very little instruction in order to read. But not all GLPs are hyperlexic. How do we support them? The rest of this chapter is devoted to providing quality literacy supports that are tailored to the needs of GLPs.

It is never too late to acquire literacy

The techniques and ideas in this chapter can be used with older students and even adults. Acquiring just a few basic literacy skills makes an enormous difference to a person's ability to access our world.

Who should support literacy?

Whilst the teacher will have ultimate responsibility, everyone who interacts with a child has a role to play in their literacy development. Teachers will often lack confidence in supporting non-speaking or minimally speaking children with their literacy acquisition. These students' journey into literacy will be different because they don't have the option of 'sounding out' using conventional phonics approaches. As this chapter shows, phonics is not the only route into literacy.

Literacy teaching should not be restricted to literacy lessons. It should be incorporated into every subject so that the child gets repeated opportunities to apply skills throughout the school day.

In fact, literacy comes into virtually all daily activities. Whether it is reading environmental print and pointing out the letters and sounds in packaging, logos, road signs and clothing, or writing lists and notes for everyday activities. The more a child is exposed to written text, and given opportunities to use and talk about written text, the quicker they will acquire literacy.

It may make sense to work from 'the whole' first before breaking it down

This theory is very speculative, and we will need to gather more evidence from our clinical experience, from parents and from teachers, but I wonder if we might work from the premise that GLPs begin their literacy journey from the 'whole' first. This may be a whole text, the whole sentence or a whole word. Once the GLP is familiar with the whole (and perhaps only then), they may then be ready to break it down: a whole text into sentences; a whole sentence into words; a word into phonemes or spelling patterns. I have therefore ordered the following 'first steps into literacy' in this order: the whole first (a text, a sentence, the whole alphabet), followed by steps to break it down and remix the whole (a text into sentences; a sentence into words or into 'frame-and-slot' patterns; the alphabet into groups of letters and individual letters).

First steps into literacy (in stages 1–3 of NLA)

In their book *Comprehensive Literacy for All*, Karen Erickson and David Koppenhaver set out a framework for assessing and teaching literacy.[1] The information that follows draws heavily on this work but has been adapted and re-ordered for GLPs. As with language acquisition, every GLP's journey to literacy will be highly individual. Some of these ideas may resonate; others not so much.

Early shared reading

Shared reading means enjoying texts together. This can look very different for different children, because we are starting from their interests. As always, this is a child-led experience. GLPs are led by personal meaning, emotional resonance and the richness of the whole experience. Therefore we will be watching out for the stories and texts that they are naturally drawn to.

- GLPs may need to move around when books are being read to them. This doesn't mean they are not listening: in fact being able to move around freely often helps them to listen and process.

- GLPs are likely to be drawn to books that have musical qualities: those with a repeated refrain or a rhythm, for example *We're Going on a Bear Hunt* by Michael Rosen, or any book by Julia Donaldson or Lynly Dodd.

- GLPs often enjoy quirky characters who have interesting dilemmas, take Quentin Blake's *Mrs Armitage, Queen of the Road* or *Daisy Artichoke*, or Lauren Child's 'Charlie and Lola' series.

- GLPs may enjoy audio-books in the car or before going to bed. These often have songs as part of the story, enhancing the appeal for GLPs. Repetition can be a brilliant tool in acquiring literacy. The child might 'read along' with the audio version.

- Books that have been made into animations may also be appealing: Julia Donaldson and Judith Kerr's books have recently been adapted in this way.

- Spoken word artists such as MC Grammar[2] may be appealing for older GLPs. We are looking for ways in which written text engages an individual child and appeals to their auditory preferences. If they enjoy rhythm, then choose rhythmic texts.

- GLPs who have entered stage 2 may enjoy Nick Sharratt's *Ketchup on Your Cornflakes* and *Mixed Up Fairytales*: these are perfect for modelling mitigable gestalts.

- Use a GLP's enthusiasms to guide shared reading: if they love planets, dinosaurs, vehicles, find books that involve these. Autistic children generally love to learn, and non-fiction books might be particularly appealing.

- Scholastic's 'Non-fiction sight-word readers' are brilliant for supporting stage 2: the text is arranged into 'frame-and-slots' and so a child can predict the text from the picture.

- 'Tar Heel Reader' is a wonderful website which has thousands of free online books that users have made. It is easy to search any topic, e.g. 'rainbows' or 'electricity' and find readers on this topic. The texts are also a source of potential gestalts and mitigations. Many languages are included.

- 'Pictello' is a cheap and useful app for making personalised books. It is as easy as taking a few photos and adding captions.

Early writing

Early experiments with writing are creative and fun. Scribbling and drawing gradually shapes itself into writing.

- We provide a range of writing tools: pens, pencils, crayons, chalks, markers, finger paint, sand, alphabet sets and so on.

- A small whiteboard is a particularly useful tool which can be used by both the GLP and communication partners to draw and write phrases during natural interactions and play.

- Early writing attempts look like scribble, but this is still valid. Gradually, this starts to look like lines or swirls, and then letter-like shapes begin to be grouped together.

- GLPs may show a preference for either upper-case or lower-case letters: go with their preference in early writing.

- An onscreen keyboard and a paper-based alphabet chart are also options. At first, the letter selections will be random, just as a child with a pencil will scribble. Gradually though, letters might be grouped together into word shapes.

- We might offer 'predictable chart writing' for children who have arrived at stage 2. We can write out their mitigated gestalt and offer other options. For example, for a child who is mitigating from 'what do you see? I see a . . .' we might swop in words like 'brown bear', 'green frog' or even 'purple dinosaur'.

- Stage 3 GLPs may enjoy telling adults what to write and draw. We can label pictures that a child has drawn to help them make the association between the written word and the referent.

- Word tiles or word labels may be appealing for GLPs who are in stage 3. They could match these to items or pictures.

Exposure to the alphabet and phonological awareness

GLPs will have a tendency to learn the whole alphabet first, often through the alphabet song. They may not want to separate out the letters until they are well into stage 2. We respect this.

- Once a GLP has started breaking down the alphabet, they may be more receptive to activities where letters are found in isolation, for example, finding letters buried in sand, using letter cookie cutters with playdough.

- GLPs may like having a familiar line such as 'a is for apple' for each letter. When they are securely in stage 2, they may be receptive to other options: 'a is for alligator' and so on.

- A stage 3 GLP may enjoy alphabet books, or making their own book of pictures starting with the first letter in their name.

- Regarding phonics teaching, having a song for each phoneme can be a way to engage a stage 1–3 GLP. Twinkl have a good resource for this, where there is a slide for the phoneme and a suggested song, using the tune of a familiar song. Search for 'phonics mnemonics songs' if you have a Twinkl account.

- However bear in mind that a stage 1–3 GLP will be unlikely to be able to encode or decode words from phonics instruction.

- GLPs are more likely to acquire literacy through 'whole word recognition', or even a 'whole sentence' approach. It is helpful for GLPs to see us writing down their gestalts and mitigations. We may do this using pen and paper, on a whiteboard or typing them on an iPad, throughout the day.

- It is also helpful for GLPs to see us writing down lines from songs or books, and writing down steps in an instruction.

- For GLPs in stage 3 and above, we can write lists of things: shopping lists, packing lists, lists of children's names and so on.

- Rhyme awareness and alliteration may be explored through songs and books. GLPs who are in the early stages of NLA are unlikely to be able to make sense of rhyme matching games, and so they should simply be exposed to songs and books using these features, rather than being expected to complete a task.

Conventional literacy teaching (in stages 4–6 of NLA)

Once a child

1. knows most of the letters of the alphabet most of the time,

2. engages in shared reading,

3. has a means of communication and

4. understands that print carries meaning

then they are ready to move on to 'conventional' literacy teaching. This is probably going to also require a child to be in stage 4 of NLA, as they will need to answer questions, as well as be able to create self-generated sentences.

Conventional literacy teaching includes phonics, spelling patterns, reading comprehension and writing a range of different texts. Each of these elements is explored in more detail next.

Synthetic versus analytic phonics

GLPs do not naturally segment words and 'sound out'. Therefore synthetic phonics, the dominant way of teaching early literacy in the UK, will be challenging. Synthetic phonics is where a word is made up of each separate phoneme, e.g. 'sh – i – p', 'b – a – ck'. However there is also something called analytic phonics, and this may be more accessible, because it makes use of visual spelling patterns. In this approach, words can be collected into 'word families' based on their spelling pattern, e.g. m-ake, c-ake, t-ake, b-ake, r-ake. This is also known as 'rime-and-onset'.

Rime-and-onset word families lend themselves to visual games where the first letter (the onset) is detachable from the rest of the word (the rime). We can show this visually by having a brick with the onset written on it, e.g. 'h', and another brick with the rime written on it, e.g. 'en'. This spells 'hen'. We can then show that the first brick can be swopped with different onset letters, e.g. 'p', 'm', 'd' and that this makes different words: 'pen', 'men', 'den'.

Exactly the same principle applies with a range of media. We could write different onsets on one half of a plastic egg and the rime on the other half. If you turn one half of the egg, the word changes. If you search 'word family craft ideas' online you can see some brilliant ideas: two paper cups, one inside the other with a cut-out window; plates shaped like flowers with different petal rimes and so on.

Spelling patterns

The most common spelling patterns in English are shown in Table 13.1. Systematic teaching of each of these spelling patterns will allow a child to read at least 500 words.

Table 13.1 The most common spelling patterns in English

ack	ail	ap	ash	aw	ale	ake
ate	ay	ank	an	ain	ame	all
eat	ell	ice	ide	it	ick	ip
ight	ill	in	ing	op	ot	oke
ore	ock	uck	ug	ump	est	ink
at	unk					

Words might be sorted into their word families, for example – ay and – unk words. Later, the child might be asked to generate words for a word family when they are given the rime. An alphabet chart or onscreen keyboard can be used for this.

Sight words

Sight words are high-frequency words which often have irregular spellings and cannot be sounded out, e.g. 'the', 'you', 'was', 'are'. GLPs will have been exposed to sight words in their 'emergent' literacy, through whole sentence reading. Now, if they have reached stage 4 in their spoken language, they will be able to segment the sentence and process these words as single units.

It can be helpful to have a systematic order for learning sight words, with regular revision built in. A 'word wall' might be built to reflect the sight words that have been learnt. Lists of sight words by year-group are available online.

GLPs who have strong visual processing may be able to pick up sight words simply through regular reading for pleasure and exposure to text through media. Reading in context may make more sense for GLPs than reading from a list or a word wall: we will need to have an individualised approach to literacy, just as we did for their language acquisition.

Independent reading

Children are more likely to engage with books if they have completely free choice of reading material.

- This may be picture books, story books, factual books, magazines, comics, online books, or even catalogues, websites and videos with captions. Use their enthusiasms to search for titles they may enjoy.

- The child may choose a text which is either way below or way above their current reading level. This is ok: the adult can still support their reading attempts of the text.

- For GLPs who are in stage 4 or above, conversation around what they did or didn't enjoy can be part of the reading experience.

- The child can be encouraged to follow the text with an adult. If it is an online book, the text being spoken might be highlighted. This encourages independent reading, and reading for pleasure.

- GLPs often enjoy watching tv with the subtitles on. Allow them to do this where possible.

Reading should take place in a space where the child is comfortable and their sensory needs are being met.

Reading for learning

Autistic children love learning. We can make use of their enthusiasms here. We might set them a challenge question to find out new information from a piece of text. For example, 'which is the biggest planet?' or 'why do we see colours in a rainbow?' It is important that the question is engaging and has the right degree of challenge for an individual.

Writing for sharing

GLPs will probably be motivated to write about their enthusiasms. We can encourage them to find or make interesting images around their enthusiasms, and then to create text to accompany these. Starter questions like 'if you could go anywhere, where would it be?' or 'if you were an animal, what would you be?' might be helpful.

It is helpful to establish a culture of 'writing without worrying'. First drafts should be free from rules about spelling, grammar and punctuation. If we can't read the text, we ask the child to read it back to us, and make a note of what they said. We comment on the content and not the form of the writing, e.g. 'I've learnt something new about cacti today'. This demonstrates to the child that their writing is meaningful and valued.

Writing does not have to involve a pencil. We know that many autistic children have fine motor challenges. They may access the alphabet through a letter board or a keyboard. Software such as Clicker and Docs Plus[3] give additional learning tools such as access to 'word banks' and mind-maps to organise their work.

Literacy across the curriculum

If we have arrived at this stage, GLPs are well on their way to achieving full literacy. We will continue to use their enthusiasms in literacy instruction. We will continue to use the principles of 'Universal Design'[4] to allow them to thrive in education.

Literacy will now be woven into all learning experiences, across the curriculum. It will have practical applications in daily life: writing lists, reminders and notes, writing text messages or emails, and searching for information around particular topics. We will have opened a door into independent learning, allowing our GLP to pursue their interests and enthusiasms, and ultimately to access the world around us.

The role of text-to-speech AAC

Some GLPs, particularly those who are hyperlexic, are able to access text-to-speech AAC with minimal literacy instruction.[5] Other autistic people, particularly those with dyspraxia, will need many hours of support and practice in order to reliably access the alphabet for spelling.[6]

Many autistic children begin with a symbol-based AAC system which includes an onscreen keyboard. They very naturally move over to text-to-speech because they find typing quicker than using a symbol-based AAC package.

We encourage the use of an onscreen keyboard and spelling because this gives access to unlimited AAC language. A symbol-based vocabulary package will only ever have access to a few thousand words. A truly flexible grammar is challenging in a symbol-based AAC system. We are always ultimately aiming for literacy, and therefore a text-to-speech AAC system.

All writing activities described in this chapter can be accessed using a spelling chart, keyboard or onscreen keyboard.

Summary of literacy supports

- Try working from the 'whole' first: the whole experience of exploring books, and making this appealing for the individual child. They may need to move; they may need a particular cosy space to explore a book; they may like tactile or auditory qualities in books.

- Think about the whole experience of text in our environment (logos, menus, posters, subtitles, multi-sensory play with letters and sounds). How can this be presented playfully for this child?

- Consider that a GLP may learn to read a whole sentence or a whole word before they are able to access phonics.

- Use the child's enthusiasms and interests as the entry point into literacy. Explore texts around their interests, be it sparkly objects, holes, power networks, rainbows, octopuses, recycling. . . .

- Consider the stage of NLA that the child is largely operating within. Which texts lend themselves to language development at this stage? For example repeated refrains for stage 1, predictable 'frames-and-slots' for stage 2, picture dictionaries for stage 3.

- Provide a wide range of writing tools and the whole alphabet in many different forms: a whiteboard and pens, magnetic letters, foam letters, letters hidden in sand or playdough, an onscreen keyboard.

- Offer 'predictable chart writing' for GLPs who are in stage 2 or beyond.

- Create books together by using images that appeal to the child. Make an alphabet book, or a book around the first letter of the child's name, or their favourite letter. Make books to tell the story of a special event or outing.

- Make use of songs. The alphabet song for a child in stage 1; fun rhymes for a child in stage 1 or 2; a song for each phoneme or spelling pattern for a child who is in stage 4 or beyond.

- Write down a child's gestalts and mitigations, their word isolations and their early phrases and sentences.

- Offer 'whole word' literacy teaching. Experiment with resources such as Scholastic's 'Non-Fiction Sight Word Readers' series.

- Once a child is ready for conventional literacy teaching, consider 'analytic phonics' using 'rime-and-onset' word families, rather than the ubiquitous 'synthetic phonics' programmes.

- Teach spelling patterns, making use of a child's strengths in spotting visual patterns.

- Teach 'sight words', building on lots of repetition of these in the context of meaningful sentences.

- Create a reason for a child to find out information from text, so that they can see the point of reading. Relate this to their natural interests and enthusiasms.

- Create opportunities for the child to share their writing with others, and to connect with others who may share their interests and enthusiasms through writing.

Tracking progress

GLPs may not follow predictable patterns in their literacy. They are very likely to suddenly surprise us by creating a whole phrase in text, or a longer word that is correctly spelled. Traditional tracking tools will not necessarily work for these children. Instead, observations of what they do in their own time will be more important. We can take photos and video of them engaging with written texts, enjoying songs and rhymes, experimenting with early writing and so on. We can transcribe what they might have spelled out using an alphabet chart, take photos of their text-to-speech AAC messages, and print out from Clicker matching or sentence sets.

Tracking progress with non-speaking or minimally speaking GLPs

Teaching staff are often very confused about how to assess a child's literacy if they are non-speaking or minimally speaking. They will not be able to 'read aloud' in the same way that a reliably speaking child can.

Non-speaking and minimally speaking GLPs can show their literacy acquisition by:

- Interacting with texts; showing enjoyment and engagement with written materials; pointing to words or phrases in response to an adult's comments or questions.

- Creating texts, using conventional writing tools, or using an alphabet chart, keyboard or onscreen keyboard.

- Matching words or sentences to pictures and objects using paper-based materials or using software such as Clicker.[7]

- Answering questions using their AAC. They might be able to say what they liked about a story, and if they are at stage 4 or above, they might be able to answer wh- questions about the text.

- To show their learning of particular letters and sounds, spelling patterns or sight words, we can offer options, and they might point to the correct one or indicate 'yes' when we point to it, e.g. 'which word says, "he"? This one? This one? This one?'

- This technique can also be used for comprehension questions, e.g. 'which animal was scared? This one? This one? This one?'

Case study: Azariah

Azariah's mum, Ebony, contacted me to ask about support for her son. Azi was 4 years old, had just been identified as autistic and was seeing a sensory integration trained Occupational Therapist.

Ebony told me in our first phone call that Azariah loved the Alphablocks, the solar system, flags and countries of the world. His interest in the solar system and planets was sparked when a cousin bought him a My First Atlas *book. Ebony then nourished this interest by buying more books around countries and flags of the world.*

We talked about the way that Azi communicated. He used a handful of phrases and some single words. As we talked, Ebony recognised my descriptions of Gestalt Language Processing. For example, Azariah recently sang the song 'Teddy Bear, Teddy Bear, You're My Friend' to his mum when they had shared a moment of connection. When he was upset, he would repeatedly say 'seven'. Ebony said that Azi often spoke quietly to himself, but it was difficult to hear what he was saying. She said he loved singing and being sung to.

Azariah loved to arrange items, especially in rainbow order. He had a very systematic brain, loving to organise and categorise, and was able to spot visual patterns and similarities.

At home, Azariah was exposed to a rich mixture of spoken and written language in English and Yoruba.

When I asked more about Azariah's interest in the alphabet, Ebony told me that he loves the alphabet in many forms: fridge magnets, foam letters in the bath and an alphabet eggs set. At nursery he made words out of Lego blocks and wooden shape pieces. He also loved it when adults wrote letters and words, and he attempted to trace over these.

Ebony also told me that Azariah could read books. Particular favourites were God Loves Me *and* Little Scientists. *Provided that there was not too much text on the page, he could pick up a book and read it without adult help.*

In our initial sessions, Azi loved playing with pretend food. He spontaneously named many food items, but also repeated some of the phrases that I used, like 'we could eat some', and 'it's delicious'. He loved arranging these items on the table, often in rainbow order, and also by category, sorting fruit from vegetables.

Azi would play with the food and then take himself to the trampoline and bounce for 30 seconds. He loved my singing to him when he did this, and gave me gorgeous eye contact and a wide smile.

In the next few sessions I also got out some alphabet toys, including an alphabet train and Alphablocks. Azi arranged the alphabet train in order, but grouping the letters in the same groups as we sing the lines in the alphabet song, e.g. 'abcdefg . . . hijklmnop . . . qrstuv . . . wxyz'. Azi then took the 'k' and put it beneath the 'c', saying [k k k] and looking at me to make sure that I understood they made the same sound.

I had some word cards that accompanied the alphabet train set, which spelled out words like 'bus', 'star' and 'frog'. Azi took these cards, where the words were spelled in uppercase letters, and used the Alphablocks to spell the words out, letter by letter. He said the name and sound of each letter as he constructed the word, and then he read the whole word back.

Azi then started to spell out his own CVC (consonant-vowel-consonant) words with the Alphablocks, switching the first letter each time, as if playing with word families. For example, 'van' became 'fan' became 'zan' became 'man'. He said each word after he had made it, and there were nonsense words as well as real words. Azi then began to make CCVC words, using a 'rime-and-onset' pattern and using his knowledge of which sound clusters are viable, e.g.

'th-an', 'sm-an', 'pl-an'. When he spelled out a real word, Azi paused and read it a few times, as if to acknowledge this.

Azi also spelled out 'sight words', showing particular interest in the word 'on'. Since I like to follow the thread of what children are exploring, I modelled some phrases using this word, both saying it and writing the phrase on a small whiteboard, e.g. 'on my head', 'on the table'. Azi was interested in what I was writing, and briefly attempted to write letters himself. He used a very strong pressure on the pen, just as he tended to use strong pressure and big movements with all toys and materials, suggesting a sensory processing component.

Azi returned to his Alphablocks word 'on', saying it to himself quietly. I got out a favourite book, Ketchup on Your Cornflakes, which has lots of different 'frame-and-slot' fun phrases which can be changed by turning the half page, e.g. 'do you like . . .' 'ketchup . . . on your head?' 'ketchup . . . in your bath?' 'toothpaste . . . on your cornflakes?' etc. Azi followed along as I pointed to the words that I was reading.

At the end of the session, I discussed hyperlexia with Ebony. She told me that he had first recited the alphabet when he was 9 months old, and used the alphabet to self-regulate. Indeed as he was putting his shoes on to go, Azi could be heard saying 'O-N-E . . . one, T-W-O . . . two'.

Over the next few sessions I offered alphabet and literacy based supports, including magnetic letters, whiteboard and pens, and books.

In one session, Azi tipped out all of the magnetic letters in a tray, and then spelled 'alphabet'. Then he added to this, spelling out 'the alphabet song'. Azi looked at me when I acknowledged what he had done. He then spelled out 'now I know' and I said, 'now I know my abc, next time won't you sing with me?' Azi looked and smiled, and then jumped on the trampoline for some excited bouncing. He came back and spelled a little more, saying each word as he spelled it. He stopped when he got to the 'n' in 'next time won-'. I offered him the 't' but he didn't want it: he was looking for an apostrophe! Fortunately, the set had punctuation marks too. Azi finished the rest of the line of the song, complete with apostrophe and question mark.

Azi made brilliant progress with our therapy sessions, acquiring lots of gestalts that were modelled. His literacy really helped with mitigations, as I could show him, through writing, using magnetic letters or typing on an AAC app, how we could switch words in and out of a sentence.

Ebony was able to explain to Azi what was going to happen by writing on a piece of paper that Azariah could hold on to. This helped him to manage transitions and changes.

Along with his interest in reading books and environmental print, Azi was well on his way to literacy, and his literacy was supporting his continued language development. This was all before he started school!

Notes

1 Erickson, K. & Koppenhaver, D. (2020) *Comprehensive Literacy for All: Teaching Students with Significant Disabilities to Read and Write* Brookes Publishing.
2 See https://www.mrmcgrammar.com/
3 See https://www.cricksoft.com/uk/clicker/
4 See https://udlguidelines.cast.org/
5 See https://thisisnotaboutme.film/ about Jordyn Zimmerman, for example.
6 See https://i-asc.org/s2c-spelling-to-communicate/ about the 'Spelling to Communicate' approach.
7 See https://www.cricksoft.com/uk/clicker/

Chapter 14

Supporting older GLPs

'To explain what friendship means to me I first must share what it is like to be alone.

Deciding to be alone is sometimes easier because I can feel when I am not truly accepted. Being with people who don't get me is just so hard. They want to, but inside they are uncomfortable, not fully able to accept me for who I am.'

Jordyn, from the short film *Jordyn's Rocky Journey*[1]

Recognising the experiences of an older GLP

Older GLPs, by which I mean older children, young people and even adults, have so much more life experience behind them. We know that GLPs have good episodic memories. They can store details that neurotypicals forget. They may recall events in granular detail from years and years ago. They have built a vast amount of information, good and bad, about the world around them and the people who may have tried (or not tried) to communicate with them.

We will need to honour the experiences of this person. We will need to be sensitive to the trauma of not being understood or recognised as a communicator. We will need to move slowly to gain trust. There may have been a deep sense of failure in the past, shared by those around the young person.

How might an older GLP present?

An older GLP may have moved through the NLA stages and be in later stages, or they may be at earlier stages.

There will be GLPs who did not naturally move through the stages of Natural Language Acquisition. They may be in stage 1. In fact, they may have stopped sharing their stage 1 language. If no one around them knew what to do with this, then this person may have stopped sharing their natural language. It may have gone 'underground'. Hopefully it is still in their heads, and we can let them know that we are now listening.

Older GLPs may

- Use a lot of rote language that has been taught to them, e.g. 'I want . . .'
- Be dependent on other people prompting them to speak.

DOI: 10.4324/9781032717029-14

- Have some 'set pieces' where they initiate communication and there is an expected response from the communication partner. They may find it distressing if the partner does not supply the required response.

- Have hundreds of single words, but these have not developed into longer phrases because they are probably 'stuck gestalts'.

- Have hundreds of longer gestalts, but have not moved into mitigating these.

- Hide their real language. They possibly have language internally but are silent. They maybe talk very quietly to themselves. They may 'hide behind' character voices and scripts.

- Prefer media clips and songs to talking. Their choice of scripts or songs may express profound observations on the world around them.

- Be extremely hesitant, if not resistant, to working with us, until we have earned their trust.

- Have profound motor challenges that prevent their bodies from carrying out intended actions.

- Be desperate to connect with us, but are unable to show this.

- Show their abilities when we give them the opportunity to express themselves, through their preferred modalities.

This is powerful (and emotional)

There are emotional challenges for everyone involved when we work with a young person or an adult who has not had the best support to develop their natural language. The people around this person were likely doing their very best, with the knowledge that they had. We have all made mistakes in the past, and we all have regrets about people we have known and cared about. As therapists or parents, this is highly distressing.

There may be scenarios where an autistic child or young person is signed up to programmes that we find problematic. Sometimes we stay involved because we know that this person desperately needs one person in their life who 'gets it', and we believe that we can model a better way. Sometimes we have to state clearly that our approach is incompatible with another behaviourist approach. We will need to seek professional supervision and support. We will have to examine our own values and ethics and think about how we best approach the situation.

Even when everyone involved is on the same page, there is pressure when we are working with an older GLP. We are all desperate for this to work. We will need to be even more aware of our own emotional regulation, and aware of what others are bringing into the mix. We need to work at staying in the moment, and prioritising connection with this young person.

We may consider training to become more trauma-informed. If the person has experienced behavioural approaches that have not affirmed their neurodivergence, harm has been done. We will need to be alert to potential triggers. It may be a big step for a person to simply share their space with us.

All children crave connection

All children, young people and adults crave connection. As soon as we have recognised this, we have made a momentous step. There is no such thing as 'pre-intentional'. All conscious human beings need and want connection. All conscious human beings are communicating. Some are communicating in conventional ways, and others in unconventional ways that may be more difficult to recognise and interpret. This does not mean that the will is not there.

It's never too late

As soon as we recognise that a child is a communicator, we change their life for the better. Of course, parents were there long before we were. We have been guilty of not believing parents who have told us 'he/she understands everything'. Now we can do better.

Our belief will inevitably influence others who surround that child. Now we are all listening, watching and readying ourselves for connection.

There used to be a belief that grammatical development stops at a certain point in a child's life. Marge Blanc's research[2] involved children who came to NLA at 6–9 years of age, and they could still move through stages 1–4. Research is needed for older GLPs, but there is no reason at present to believe that older children and young people cannot continue to make progress.

Horizontal development

There is enormous value in just recognising a child is a communicator. We will change their experience of the world by acknowledging their unconventional modes of communication: their stimming, their sensory or motor experiences, the objects or images they are drawn to, the photographs they take, the media they consume.

A GLP will benefit enormously from being supported in stage 1 if they have never experienced this support previously. For the first time their communication is valued and validated.

A GLP who does not have reliable speech, is non-speaking or minimally speaking can join us in experiments with AAC. Their individuality will drive innovation and creativity. We only have to take a first step. AAC is trial-and-error: we do not need the entire solution from the outset, just some options (see Chapter 12).

A GLP will have access to many more communication opportunities if we support them to move into stage 2. The move from stage 1 to stage 2 is any change from the original gestalt: trimming it down, using a 'frame-and-slot' variation or mix-and-matching different chunks.

People treat a stage 2 communicator very differently compared with a stage 1 communicator. Many more people are now able to 'get them'.

Even if they never move any further, there is a wealth of language to explore in stage 2. It is almost limitless. Stage 2 gives them access to many more communication partners and communication contexts.

The subtle art of supporting older GLPs

Our work with older GLPs is likely to be more nuanced and require a higher level of observation and reflection. We will need to think about themes in their play, movement and sensory choices, or topics of communication. What are they trying to tell us? Their meaning may sometimes be obscure (to us) and require some detective work. We will earn trust and respect by putting in the thinking time, and making educated guesses. Sometimes we'll get it right, sometimes the message will elude us. Fortunately all GLPs whom I have worked with have been extremely forgiving.

We give space and silence

A GLP who has experienced compliance-based interventions, or a GLP who has not been well understood will need time in order to start to trust us. We will need to keep our distance initially. We may need to expand our peripheral attention, not directly gazing at them, but at what they are interested in. We need to show them that we are not going to interfere or change what they are doing.

We may take a lot of non-verbal turns. A nod of the head or a 'mmm' may be enough. We are sensitive to this person's possible history of prompted language.

Respecting their age and maturity

Where we might be exuberant and expressive with younger GLPs, older GLPs may appreciate a more subdued communication style. We don't want to patronise or irritate by being too loud or too gushing. As with all GLPs, we want our language to be appealing: we will need to take into account the young person's age and experience. We also need to be our authentic selves: we don't want to try too hard! If we realise that we have overstepped the mark, we will acknowledge this and modify our approach.

We will want to match our turns to theirs. If anything, our turns should be shorter. An older GLP may have had experience of compliance-based therapy. It may take a while for them to trust that we are not trying to impose language on them. We don't want them to tune us out as background noise.

Energy shifts

It will be helpful to get to know this person's tempo. We tend to have a natural pace and rhythm. Some people are naturally slower paced and more at the relaxed end of the continuum; others are naturally at the active and sensory-seeking end of the continuum. This is where working with an Occupational Therapist trained in sensory integration may be of immense help: they may be able to advise on how to help calm or alert a person so that they are in a receptive and regulated place.

When we know this person well, we will be able to notice when the energy shifts. When their body language, their pace, their volume, voice quality, the intensity of concentration or focus changes. This is likely to be when we most need to observe and listen, and stay quiet. We are providing co-regulation.

Older GLPs are likely to be very aware of our emotional regulation and our joint attention. They know when we 'get them'. They know when we are joining them in their world and when we are being present and 'in the moment' with them. Our authenticity is crucial.

Privacy versus safeguarding

We need to take careful consideration of an older GLP's right to privacy. We will need to carefully consider the details that we share with others. If we have established trust, we do not want to jeopardise this with careless sharing. We are open with what we do need to share in the case of a safeguarding situation.

Older GLPs are likely to have excellent episodic memory. We may not. It will be helpful to take notes of significant themes, and to show the person that we remember what they have communicated with us. We can apologise when we forget and need a reminder.

Qualitative analysis of language samples

Our language samples may be more informative in their qualitative rather than quantitative information. We may be less interested in percentages of utterances in different stages than the variety of language in a stage. We will be interested in variety of form and function: the range of vocabulary and phrase structures, and the range of communication intentions.

An older GLP who has a lot of media scripts, particularly from movies or tv programmes, may take on different voices or characters. They may find it easier to express certain emotions or thoughts when they are in character. It will be helpful for us to get to know these films and characters. We may need to do a bit of background research by watching them!

Modes of communication

It is never too late to introduce AAC. If previous attempts have not been successful, we may need to start from scratch, using GLP principles. We need to explore literacy as an option (see Chapter 13). It is always possible that a GLP is hyperlexic, or has acquired literacy without this having been fully recognised.

There are many potential modalities: symbolised or text-to-speech AAC, writing or drawing, or taking photos. Many older GLPs are drawn to visual arts. Looking back at their choice of images or constructions can be highly regulating. We might consider helping to make a portfolio of work, with images accompanied by potential stage 1 and 2 language. Music, art or drama therapy may be transformative for this individual.

Supporting transition into other settings

When a child or young person is transitioning into new educational, work or recreational settings, we will want to make supporting adults aware of their communication preferences and potential. We may make a communication passport with the GLP, in their chosen modality. For example, they may have a paper-based, digital or video communication passport. They should have ownership over information they wish to share.

The way that we interact with this person is profound. It communicates powerfully to others this person's competence and autonomy. This is setting the precedent for future interactions, for future relationships. We are establishing the cultural values for our community.

Liaison with families

We are more likely to be supporting older GLPs in school, and so the link with home is really important. We might schedule regular catch-ups with parents or carers so that we are each aware of any developments in the GLP's communication, and what they are choosing to access during leisure time. For instance, are there any technologies, apps or games that the GLP is enjoying? They might have discovered online shopping, or Google maps, or creating images using AI. They may be accessing an interest group around their enthusiasms. They may like going to specific shops or amusement parks or exhibitions in the school holidays. This knowledge can provide inspiration for our sessions with them.

The language of identity and self-advocacy

Self-advocacy is the ability to express our wants, needs, preferences and rights. It requires others to listen and respect those choices. Self-advocacy is very much intertwined with power relationships and privilege. The more marginalised identities a person holds, the less likely they are to be encouraged to self-advocate.

We need to be aware of this, and build this into our therapy. Autistic and neurodivergent people are in the neurominority, and their needs are easily overlooked by the neuromajority. If we add in any other marginalised identities, this will be exacerbated: if they are not white; if they have a learning disability; if they are not straight or do not have a binary gender expression.

Increasingly there are free resources to help us explore identity and self-advocacy. We might explore websites such as 'Autistic Self-Advocacy Network', 'Ambitious about Autism' and 'Autism in Black'.

This is work for our whole culture. We have an important role as allies. Everything we do, write, portray and share is important in raising this issue. We can change the narrative around neurodiversity, autism, disability and intersectionality. Every conversation we have, every email we write, every report we write, every time we question or challenge current practice is an opportunity for changing the status quo.

Some useful questions that we might use and model are:

- Why is it done this way?

- Where did that come from?

- Who does that serve?

- Is that fair?

- Is it time to change this?

Summary of supports for older GLPs

- Believe in them as communicators. We assume competence for all human beings, including those who have learning disabilities.

- Respect what they are trying to tell us, even when they are using unconventional modalities.

- Introduce AAC where it is needed. It is never too late to start.

- Observe the themes in their play, their sensory or motor patterns, and their language.

- Make sensitive attempts to interpret what they are trying to communicate. We acknowledge when we have not quite got it right.

- Be aware of the length of our turns, our volume and style of talking, our animation, our tempo.

- Be aware of shifting energy: body language, pace, volume, intensity of purpose.

- Be silent when it matters: when they are trying to tell us something important.

- Research their favourite tv programmes, movies and characters in order to reach a deeper understanding of what they might mean to the GLP.

- Talk to their families about their activities at home. What technologies do they access? What games or apps do they choose? How do they choose to engage with their environment and community?

- Be sensitive to previous experiences of this person, including compliance-based therapy and possibly trauma.

- Consider the role of other therapies, e.g. sensory integration, music, art or drama therapy.

- Provide the language of self-advocacy, in terms of needs and preferences, bodily sensations and possible regulatory supports.

- Support transition to other settings and contribute to a culture that values and validates all communication.

- Contribute to a different dialogue around the needs of the neurominority.

- Draw attention to the intersection of neurodivergence and marginalised identities and ask questions in order to drive policy changes in schools, workplaces and society.

Case study: Ashok

Ashok's dad contacted me about supporting his son's spoken language. He was specifically wondering how we could support him to become more conversational. He recognised that Ashok used a lot of scripting based on things he had read and songs that he listened to. Ashok's parents wondered how they could find a way into this language in order to connect meaningfully.

We arranged for me to meet Ashok, aged 10 years old, in school. He came with his teacher to his first session. Ashok enjoyed a race-track that I had brought and used mitigations such as 'the red car is winning!' and 'the purple car is winning!' There was also evidence of stage 3 and stage 4 language, with words being used fairly flexibly in constructions such as 'game!', 'game over', 'play the game?' and 'this game'. He also clearly loved the alphabet and numbers, ordering them correctly and singing songs associated with them. Ashok showed me that he was able to read, reading the text on the boxes of toys.

As I got to know Ashok, I recognised that he often came into our sessions in a dysregulated or excited state. He would use an almost painfully loud voice. I had to stay completely quiet, or if I needed to talk, I had to use a calm, low voice for the first ten minutes or so. Ashok would then reduce his volume and appear more settled. Ashok loved any resources that involved solving problems, using numbers or playing with alphabet letters. He loved to sing, but hated it if I tried to join in.

As I took language samples, I found that he was using language from a mixture of stages, but that he would perhaps benefit from more variety in stage 2 in order to provide material for later stages. I shared my language samples and notes from each session with his teacher and parents, and sent short video clips to his parents so that they could see the supports in action as we played and interacted.

Since Ashok loved to read, I brought in books that I thought might interest him. He became absorbed in some of my choices; for others he would toss them aside. I modelled language around this, e.g. 'I don't like this one' and 'that's not interesting'.

At home Ashok was now accessing tv with the subtitles switched on. His parents reported that he loved to draw and he was beginning to label his drawings with captions. He would draw vehicles or buildings with comments like 'stand back, train approaching' or 'lift going up'. In our sessions, Ashok used magnetic letters to spell out the names of brands like 'Costa' and 'Smiths Toys' and signs that he had seen, e.g. 'Shell Recharge' and 'Deli Go'.

At each school holiday I arranged an online meeting with Ashok's parents. They shared with me what he was seeking out in his leisure time. He was enjoying browsing his favourite sweets and desserts on the Sainsbury's website, and was also using Google Maps to look up the location of his favourite shops, supermarkets and petrol stations.

It was invaluable to know what Ashok was seeking out spontaneously, as I could incorporate these interests into our sessions.

Taking inspiration from his parents reporting that Ashok liked Google Maps, I brought in an atlas and some travel guides. Ashok showed me that he already knew a lot about countries and flags, and so I made a game where we could match flags. I wondered if Ashok was beginning to experiment with stage 3 language, as he would isolate the name of the flag from my phrases. For example, I would say 'I think it's Poland', and he said 'Poland' or 'not Poland . . . Indonesia!'

I had an app where we could build a town, adding in features like supermarkets, playgrounds and cafes. This provided opportunities for more stage 2 language like 'how about a road here?' and 'how about more shops?'

I brought in games around shopping and going to the café. Ashok showed me that he already had language around these activities, saying 'two scoops?' and 'some sprinkles!' I took his language and remixed it, and he did the same, showing me that he was able to build stage 4 word + word + word novel utterances, e.g. 'more rainbow sprinkles' and 'want caramel scoop?' when he was well-regulated.

I knew that school was a challenging sensory environment for Ashok. He did not like the loud hustle and bustle of a classroom, and often chose a quieter reading area instead. I also realised, when watching back a video of one of our sessions, that the fluorescent light in the school therapy room looked like it was flashing on and off. This could have been contributing to Ashok's initial dysregulation. Being a typical therapy room cupboard in a school, it was dark if I turned the light off. Another therapist who I supervise mentioned that she brings in her own disco ball light to her sessions. I wondered if I could try a more natural portable light, and to my delight I found a lamp shaped like a globe. This helped both of us with our regulation, and provided another source of language, as we turned the globe and talked about countries, continents, oceans and mountains.

I noticed that I needed to be flexible in the stage of language I was consciously supporting. Ashok's stage of language modulated within a session, perhaps depending upon his regulation, mood and creative impulses. In one session, he might come in and sing his favourite songs very loudly (I had to cover my ears for this!) but after a few minutes, he would settle into some stage 2, 3 or 4 language. I had to engage my best listening, trying to get a sense of where he was at, and then I might offer a smattering of language in response. I think Ashok particularly appreciated my quiet turns: I had learnt by now that he was a thoughtful, reflective personality. It felt calming to just be together, with no pressure for either of us to 'perform'. And of course if I just let a session unfold, he would often surprise me with a new grammatical construction or new vocabulary.

At our next catch-up, Ashok's mum said that she was noticing that he was becoming more interactive in his language use. He was using vocabulary she had never heard from him before, like 'that's disgusting!' or 'it's frozen'. He was now asking questions and waiting for the answer. If he didn't like the answer he might say 'that's not right' or 'no, not that'. She could then model language like 'we can't go to Sainsbury's today' or 'have to wait for more pocket money'. Whilst Ashok did not always like this, he did appear to understand it, and there was a reduction in his becoming dysregulated when his wishes were thwarted.

The school environment continued to be challenging for Ashok, and I knew that I still had work to do in helping him advocate for himself. He was very much at risk of being labelled with 'challenging behaviour': he was becoming a strong and tall young man, who occasionally had emotional outbursts. He did not always understand personal space, and could not always control his impulse to reach out and grab. His changing body was perhaps exacerbating everything.

Thinking about this made me explore resources around regulation and interoception, as well as considering social stories which offered options. I knew that I had an important role in influencing the narrative around Ashok. As we enter the next school year, I will be exploring these advocacy tools with his teaching team.

Notes

1 See https://jordynsrockyjourney.wordpress.com/
2 Blanc, M. (2012) *Natural Language Acquisition on the Autism Spectrum: The Journey from Echolalia to Self-Generated Language* Madison, WI: Communication Development Center, Inc.

Chapter 15

Neurodiversity-affirming practice

Taking responsibility

As a profession, we are responsible for many of the misconceptions and outdated practices surrounding autism. We didn't know any better then, but we do now.

We need to listen to autistic people. They are the best judges of helpful and unhelpful approaches. They have educated us in the last few years and allowed us to recognise that it is not ok to try to make them look neurotypical. In their paper 'Autistic Self-Advocacy and the Neurodiversity Movement', Leadbitter et al state that

> **all autism intervention stakeholders need to understand and actively engage with the views of autistic people and with neurodiversity as a concept and movement. In so doing, intervention researchers and practitioners are required to move away from a normative agenda and pay diligence to environmental goodness-of-fit, autistic developmental trajectories, internal drivers and experiences, and autistic prioritized intervention targets.[1]**

We need to talk to one another and educate one another. We need to challenge ourselves and one another if we have a hunch that what we are doing is not right. We need to be brave and admit our mistakes and knowledge gaps. It is ok to have made mistakes in the past, but to continue to do so when updated information is available is not ok.

Neurodiversity-affirming language

We need to change the language that we use around autism. Since autism was first identified, it has been associated with judgemental language from a neurotypical perspective that has simply compared autistic individuals with neurotypical individuals and concluded that autistic individuals are the ones with the deficits. This is gradually changing, and as a profession we need to do our bit.

DOI: 10.4324/9781032717029-15

We cannot reference ALP norms with GLP children and young people

We need to stop writing reports which compare GLPs with ALP norms for eye contact, attention and listening, receptive language and expressive language. Autistic children follow different patterns and trajectories of development. By continuing to use neurotypical norms for neurodivergent children we are demonstrating and perpetuating the 'double empathy problem'.[2]

The 'double empathy problem'

Damian Milton[3] coined this term to describe how it is difficult for autistic people to interpret neurotypical patterns of behaviour and communication, and it is equally difficult for allistic (non-autistic) people to interpret neurodivergent patterns of behaviour and communication. Because allistic people are the 'neuro-majority', we have dominated the narrative around strengths and deficits, and around empathy. But we are equally lacking in understanding and empathy when it comes to autistic culture. We have assumed that the neuro-majority culture is the 'right' way to do things. Now we must be open to learning about autistic culture. We can only learn this from autistic people. In short, we need to listen to autistic voices. When writing our reports or making notes, we need to observe, and not judge. We need to describe what we see and hear, using neutral (or positive) language.

Eye contact

The apparent lack of eye contact in autism has been overstated in our profession. Many autistic adults prefer adapted face-watching, or connecting closely with communication partners using different modalities.

We do experience spontaneous eye contact when we connect with autistic children. Perhaps we are more likely to see eye contact when a child is regulated, respected and an equal partner in an interaction. Autistic children are profoundly sensitive to the attitudes of their communication partners. If we prioritise connection and assume competence, we may see a different pattern of eye contact, along with other non-verbal communication patterns.

Non-verbal communication

It now mystifies me that as a profession we have not honoured 'hand-leading' as intentional communication. Of course, hand-leading is intentional communication: just as valid as vocalisation, reaching and eye-pointing.

Stimming too can be a means of communication. Neurotypicals may be much less adept at reading 'stimming': whether it is joyful stimming or regulating stimming, but we can learn to read this powerful non-verbal communication. Parents, once again, can help us to interpret different stims for a particular child. For example, a parent has described to me how her child uses the different 'toots' from Thomas trains, and these indicate his mood. The Thomas toot is his happy noise, whilst the Gordon toot is his grumpy noise.

Attention and listening

Attention and listening is different in autism. Autistic children do not have to look in order to listen. To our neurotypical bias, they may look like they are not attending, but they are. Their ability to reproduce chunks of language after the event, sometimes months or years afterwards, would suggest that their attention and listening is pretty good!

Accounts from autistic adults inform us that there are often asynchronies between different sensory modalities, a topic which is explored in a recommended paper by Pat Amos.[4] Where neurotypicals perceive the sight and sound of a person speaking as synchronous, autistic people may not (neurotypicals can get a sense of this when the audio of a movie becomes out of time with the video). A solution to this is to cut out one modality: to look away from the person speaking, in order to listen in.

Autistic people describe being able to feel an intense joy in sensory and physical experiences, patterns and wholes, that often elude neurotypicals. Maybe we neurotypicals would be distracted if we were able to see rainbows in water droplets or hear an individual bird's song within environmental noise.

In a review of the literature around autism and attention, Gernsbacher et al[5] describe how autistic children use 'covert attention' and peripheral vision to attend to what is happening in a room. They also describe how autistic children may experience 'gaze dyspraxia' where they struggle to turn to a visual stimuli, particularly when directed to by an adult. They conclude their review by advising adults to reduce demands on autistic children's attention and instead follow their focus of interest, in order to enhance connection and interaction.

Receptive language

We do not currently have any way of assessing receptive language in stages 1 and 2 of NLA. Our information-carrying words (or key-words) informal assessments are not appropriate for GLPs. We can only speculate about receptive language based on our observations and our language samples. These are so unique and individual that I cannot imagine a formal or informal assessment that would be able to compare one GLP with a larger group of GLPs (though that might well be my lack of imagination!).

Until there is such an assessment, the least harmful assumption is that autistic children understand well. We presume competence. I have had enough surprises in my practice to make me confident that GLPs have a vast and extensive understanding of language and social communication, which is at least as advanced as their ALP peers, and probably has many nuances in advance of them. GLPs seem to have superior ability to make connections between experiences, noting the visual, auditory and other sensory similarities. They show a beautiful creativity in their observations, noticing patterns more readily than ALP peers. There may be a higher incidence of synaesthesia (connections between one sense and another, for example seeing words in colours; feeling sounds in physical sensations).

Expressive language

Language samples are our way of tracking expressive language, but receptive language is implied. It is somewhat artificial to separate receptive and expressive language, and I choose to use the heading 'Language Acquisition' in my written reports instead of these two separate headings.

From taking language samples, we can see the variety of language a child is using and their likely communication intentions. We can state the NLA stages of language that the child is using, and give examples for these stages. We can calculate and track the relative percentages of utterances in each stage. We may choose to add further information, depending on the audience for the report or tracking tool (see the 'tracking progress' sections in the previous chapters for each of the NLA stages).

Social communication

Related to the 'double empathy problem' we need to acknowledge that our previous assumptions about autistic social communication were very flawed. In autistic-only spaces, autistic people do not have any difficulties making friends or keeping friends. Neurotypical patterns on communication may be confusing, but it is not just the responsibility of autistic people to try to make this cross-cultural awareness explicit. We should all be committed to increasing our cultural competence, and learning about autistic culture from autistic adults.

Autistic people tell us that neurotypical patterns of communication can be deeply confusing because neurotypicals do not say what they mean. In contrast autistic people are generally far more honest and direct. This is a great example of where neurotypical people may learn from autistic people, and experience more authentic, genuine communication as a result.

Autistic people are also often very aware of emotional resonances in the room. Perhaps neurotypical people are more concerned with their own performance or their own agenda, and this makes us less receptive to the subtleties of energy and emotion from others. Most parents of autistic children report that their autistic child is the first to notice if something is 'off' in the family. Also that they are the child most able to be in the moment, and able to connect with 'joy'.

It is probably helpful to note in our reports how a child best connects with another person. We can ask parents questions like: 'what do you love about your child?', 'how does your child share joy with you?', 'who connects well with your child and how do they do this?' and 'what does your child need in order to thrive?'

Sample report

The reports in the handouts section show how we might structure a more neurodiversity-affirming report. As we learn more, and start to address the double empathy problem, our report-writing will no doubt evolve.

How do we decide whether an approach is neurodiversity-affirming?

We need to engage our critical reasoning to assess whether a particular approach is neurodiversity-affirming. Some approaches are fairly obviously neurodiversity-affirming. I would put Intensive Interaction in this bracket. Many approaches, such as Hanen, are being updated to reflect current neurodiversity-affirming practice. For other approaches, it is nuanced: it depends on the interpretation. Parent-Child Interaction Therapy or VERVE Therapy would generally be considered neurodiversity-affirming where we are providing silence for regulation, but not where we are looking for neurotypical patterns of eye contact.

The definition of neurodiversity-affirming will likely evolve, but currently I would include the following features:

- Neurodivergent people value the approach.

- It celebrates autistic strengths.

- It respects the way neurodivergent people think and learn and does not try to change this.

- It does not aim to teach neurotypical patterns of communication. It values autistic identity and autistic culture.

- Multi-modal communication is celebrated and nurtured.

- It allows for unrestricted access to regulatory supports.

- It embraces and utilises individual enthusiasms and special interests.

- It empowers autistic children to advocate for their needs.

- Autistic people have input into the development of the approach, or the evolution of the approach, and their feedback has informed the updated model.

The most important of these points are those about listening to neurodivergent voices. We can learn together, be respectful of our differences, but ultimately we prioritise the experience of an autistic child. If they are not enjoying the therapy, if it is not helping them to be their authentic neurodivergent selves, then it is not an approach we should be using.

I will focus on a few autism approaches that I think need our special attention.

Applied Behavioural Analysis (ABA)

ABA developed from the Lovaas Method, which used punishment and reinforcement to eliminate undesirable autistic 'behaviours' and replaced them with desirable neurotypical behaviours. ABA aimed to suppress stimming, sensory-seeking and echolalia. It aimed to eliminate anything that marked a child out as autistic.

ABA has been updated so that punishment is no longer used (in the early days soap or pepper were sprayed in a child's face). It still makes use of rewards to promote neurotypical behaviours and suppress natural neurodivergent behaviour. Rewards take the form of sweets or treats, including sensory rewards. This might mean that a child's sensory needs are not met until they comply with a request. From a safeguarding point of view, this is extremely problematic. The child is being trained to comply with everything and anything an adult in power requires.

Unsurprisingly, autistic adults inform us that this is not acceptable. There are multiple distressing accounts from adults describing disturbing experiences with ABA.[6,7] From sensory needs not being met, to stims and echolalia being suppressed, to language being limited to a few 'survival' phrases to request predefined items.

ABA is the ultimate compliance-based intervention. It is incompatible with neurodiversity-affirming practice, and it does not have a place in Speech and Language Therapy. ABA tutors have no training in language acquisition. They are not bad people, but they have not been educated in language acquisition. Language does not develop from operant conditioning. It might look like the child is learning language, but they are just learning a script: in this situation, when the tutor says 'x', I have to say 'y'. This does not translate into Natural Language Acquisition. It does not generalise. It suppresses the Natural Language Acquisition of these children: their natural language is ignored or discouraged.

Language is our area of expertise. This is why we have a protected title. As SLTs, we have to come out and take a position on ABA. We have to inform parents that the approach is based on incorrect assumptions about language learning, and unacceptable standards of adult behaviour towards children.

Picture Exchange Communication System (PECS)

PECS is a compliance-based approach which rewards the child for using limited predefined survival language. PECS is not a robust AAC system. A robust AAC system has the following:

- Access to a range of language functions, e.g. commenting, describing, protesting, expressing joy, expressing thoughts and feelings, self-advocacy.

- Access to core and fringe vocabulary which will grow with the child's language needs.

- Access to the alphabet to allow the child to acquire literacy skills and creative language.

The language functions (or communication intentions) offered by PECS is limited to requesting objects. PECS claims to include 'commenting' at Phase IV. Using predefined phrases 'I see a . . .' and 'I hear a . . .' is not commenting. The adult has a set answer in mind, and the child must supply it. The child is not sharing their spontaneous ideas.

PECS is based on a fundamental lack of understanding about how language develops. Language is founded on connection. Language develops alongside multimodal communication, which includes spontaneous and free use of body language, facial expressions, vocalisations, pointing and gestures which are all valued and responded to. Language emerges. It is not taught. It is highly individual, depending on the interests and experiences of the individual child. To limit a child to a handful of vocabulary items and a handful of phrase types, and at best two communication intentions is not honouring the humanity of an autistic child.

Attention Autism

Attention Autism can certainly be implemented in a neurodiversity-affirming, child-led way. A lot depends on the intentions and the goals. If the intention is to be child-led and play-based, allowing a child to engage in their unique way (which includes the option to reject and protest), and for a supporting adult to then model GLP-friendly language, then Attention Autism is compatible with Natural Language Acquisition. So long as the goals are not to teach neurotypical patterns of attention and listening and turn-taking.

Social skills programmes

Over the last 30 years there have been many published programmes aiming to teach neurotypical patterns of attention and listening, turn-taking, topic maintenance and so on. Whilst these approaches were well intentioned, they are essentially teaching children how to mask their neurodivergent natural patterns of interaction. Social skills programmes are not so obviously 'compliance-based': there are not physical rewards for carrying out an instruction, but there are clear social expectations and success criteria.

Autistic people tell us that they do not have any problems with social skills when socialising with other autistic people. There is an autistic culture that is different from neurotypical culture. Rather than trying to change autistic people's social communication, we could more usefully educate ourselves and others about the differences we need to be aware of.

Instead of social skills groups, we could facilitate an autistic child accessing social networks around their enthusiasms. This is likely to result in strong friendships and a sense of identity and community.

Many social skills programmes have incorporated some degree of self-advocacy. But why have we needed to teach this separately from the rest of the curriculum? Shouldn't it just be baked in? We are all responsible for improving the autistic experience in environments designed for neurotypicals. We need to build in universal design and institutional flexibility so that there is no need for the individual to constantly need to state their sensory or movement needs. This can be as simple as considering the acoustics of a room, the lighting, the arrangement of furniture, reducing artificial scents, having quiet space and outdoor space that can be freely accessed, adjusting schedules and timetables, allowing for home-working and being competent in supporting Augmentative and Alternative Communication (AAC). These adjustments are likely to have far greater impact than social skills programmes.

The intersection of neurodivergence with other minority identities

We need to be informed about other minority identities and cultures which intersect with neurodivergence. The experience of an autistic white male is different from the experience of an autistic black male. A cisgender female autistic person's experience is different from someone who is non-binary or gender-fluid. The best way of learning about these different experiences and perspectives is through listening to autistic voices. A very small selection of voices are: Tiffany Hammond (Fidgets and Fries), Jordyn Zimmerman, Lyric Rivera (Neurodivergent Rebel), Julia Bascombe (Just Stimming), Liz Vande Putte (Actually Autistic), Rachel Dorsey, Toren Wolf, Kala Allen Omeiza and Katherine May.

Alongside neurodiversity-affirming practice, we need to inform ourselves about identity-affirming and culturally affirming practice. If we're not in a particular minority group, we are unlikely to be aware of the issues. We can ask about experiences of support and if anything could have been done better.

We know that a high proportion of neurodivergent people also identify as LGBTQIA+ and so we need to create safe spaces in order for diverse identities to be expressed. We can look at our documentation and the pronouns or the gendered terms we use. It is important that children see themselves represented in our picture books, toys and resources.

It is completely valid to include education about neurodiversity and intersectionality in our recommendations for schools and EHCPs. The more that minority voices are heard, the sooner we can provide more equitable experiences for the people we support.

How do we take this into schools?

Everything that we do or say is important. Other professionals pick up on the language we use and the attitudes that come across in our non-verbal communication. When we talk about neurodiversity using up-to-date language, we spread the word.

Here are some other ways in which we can influence practice in schools:

- We present neurodiversity-affirming practice, including NLA, as a way to increase joyful practice rather than adding to the teaching staff's 'to do' list. They will need to plan less and test less. They will connect more, play more, observe more and see natural progress.

- We note examples of best practice when we see it in classrooms. We encourage teachers to make links with one another.

- We use appreciative inquiry when we see good practice. How did they know to do this? How did they find this resource? What effect has it had?

- We provide education about Gestalt Language Processing. We model ways of interacting with GLPs in the classroom environment. We take into consideration their NLA stage and set expectations accordingly. A stage 1 or 2 GLP cannot be expected to follow an adult agenda, but they might engage with group activities if their interests and enthusiasms are incorporated. They need to move. They can't answer questions.

- We provide information about declarative language, and invite reflection about the relative value of different styles of communication and ways to track learning.

- We model how to co-regulate. We model respectful language for setting boundaries. We explain the difference between a tantrum and a meltdown.

- We offer our expertise around using a child's interests and enthusiasms in therapy, and how transformational this may be for teaching the curriculum.

- We advocate for multi-modal communication, including AAC and unconventional modes of communication.

- We model to other children in the classroom how we interact with a non-speaking child. We advocate for their needs. We speak of them with respect and admiration and highlight their strengths.

- We signpost to resources that may help with literacy, taking into consideration the child's processing style. We talk about whole-word reading, and the difference between synthetic and analytic phonics.

- We share emotional regulation and sensory regulation strategies that we have found helpful for particular children.

- We share links to resources that may be useful: examples of communication-friendly environments, seating which allows a child to move, noise-cancelling headphones, etc.

- We signpost to neurodiversity-affirming learning resources, such as the book *Just Give Him the Whale!* by Paula Kluth and Patrick Schwartz.[8]

- We signpost to Occupational Therapy for sensory integration input where needed.

- We explain the shifts in our thinking when we deliver training or write reports.

- We talk directly to the member of staff if we have concerns about a child's wellbeing because practice is not neurodiversity affirming. If needed, we take our concerns to management.

- We are clear about the reasonable adjustments that are needed in order for a child to access education.

- We use neurodiversity affirming language in our meetings, notes, therapy plans, reports and contracts with schools.

- We write detailed, specified and quantified recommendations into a child's individual plan or EHCP (Education Health Care Plan) reports.

- We recommend autistic voices to listen to in social media, podcasts, books and training.

- We learn from highly specialised educational settings and from home learning environments. Wherever neurodivergent children have been able to learn and thrive, there is information that we can use.

- We contribute to consultations from local authorities or central government. We write letters or sign petitions. We have a responsibility to share our knowledge.

As Speech and Language Therapists, we may feel that we don't hold the keys to changing the way schools work. I believe this to be outdated. As autism practitioners we are not confined to 'health'. We are very much 'education' professionals. We have a huge part to play in redefining the way that children access learning, the way their individual strengths and differences are utilised and celebrated, making a more inclusive and flexible curriculum, incorporating universal design into classrooms that benefits everyone, ensuring that learning is recognised and that some methods of assessment are not appropriate for neurodivergent children, educating adults and children about neurodiversity, and ultimately building a more inclusive society for the future.

Notes

1 Leadbitter, C., Buckle, C. L., Ellis, C. & Dekker, M. (2021, April 2) 'Autistic self-advocacy and the neurodiversity movement: Implications for autism early intervention and practice' *Frontiers in Psychology* 12.
2 Milton, D. (2012) 'On the ontological status of autism: The "double empathy problem"' *Disability and Society* 27(3), 883–887.
3 Milton, D. (2012) 'On the ontological status of autism: The "double empathy problem"' *Disability & Society* 27(6), 1–5.
4 Amos, P. (2013, April) 'Rhythm and timing in autism: Learning to dance' *Frontiers in Integrative Neuroscience* 7.
5 Gernsbacher, M., Stevenson, J., Khandakar, S. & Goldsmith, H. (2008, April) 'Why does joint attention look atypical in autism?' *Child Development Perspectives* 2(1), 38–45.
6 Kupferstein, H. (2018) 'Evidence of increased PTSD symptoms in autistics exposed to applied behavior analysis' *Advances in Autism* 4(1), 19–29.

7 McGill, O. & Robinson, A. (2020) 'Recalling hidden harms: Autistic experiences of childhood Applied Behavioural Analysis (ABA)' *Advances in Autism* 7(4), 269–282.

8 Kluth, P. & Scwartz, P. (2008) *Just Give Him the Whale! 20 Ways to Use Fascinations, Areas of Expertise, and Strengths to Support Students with Autism* Oxford Brooks Publishing.

Chapter 16

Recommended reading

The most important advice I can give to professionals or parents is to learn from autistic voices. Search out blogs, Instagram posts and websites that are created by autistic people. The ultimate test of whether an approach is neurodiversity-affirming is whether autistic people believe it to be so.

The following is a highly selective list. It includes the books that I have found most life changing and life affirming, as well as neurodiversity-affirming.

Some of these titles were released before the neurodiversity-affirming movement took off. Therefore some of the language will now strike us as outdated. However, the content is still valid.

Ido Kedar (2012) *Ido in Autismland: Climbing Out of Autism's Silent Prison*

Ido is a non-speaking autistic boy. In this memoir, he describes his experiences of being an autistic child in a world where non-speaking people are assumed to be non-thinking. He finds an AAC method that uses spelling, and is able to share his experiences with us, using beautifully poetic and nuanced language.

Naoki Higashida (2021) *The Reason I Jump: One Boy's Voice from the Silence of Autism*

Naoki is a non-speaking autistic boy. This short, poetic, easy-to-read book takes a 'question and answer' format where Naoki answers questions including 'why do you echo questions back at the asker?', 'why do you do things you shouldn't even when you've been told a million times not to?' and 'why don't you make eye contact when you're talking?'

Meghan Ashburn and Jules Edwards (2023) *I Will Die on This Hill: Autistic Adults, Autism Parents, and the Children Who Deserve a Better World*

The story of initial conflict and confusion but ultimate enlightenment and collaboration between an autistic parent and a non-autistic parent. This book highlights the importance of intersectionality in autism, and how we must consider

DOI: 10.4324/9781032717029-16

the needs of the most marginalised and minoritised autistic people in order to create a better world for everyone.

Barry Prizant (2022) *A Different Way of Seeing Autism – Revised and Expanded*

A wonderful introduction for parents and professionals to a strengths-based lens on autism. Real-life examples from families and schools, and practical strategies to make the world an easier place to negotiate for autistic people.

Julia Bascom (editor) (2012) *Autistic People, Speaking*

An eclectic and diverse mix of autistic people speaking and writing about the themes that are most important to them. This is enlightening, and at times confronting, as writers cover such topics as police brutality and aversive and abusive behavioural interventions. An important, if uncomfortable, read.

Paula Kluth and Patrick Schwartz (2008) *Just Give Him the Whale! 20 Ways to Use Fascinations, Areas of Expertise, and Strengths to Support Students with Autism*

Inspiration for teachers. How to use children's interests to foster authentic social connections; to promote self-advocacy, regulation and wellbeing; to provide joyful access to the curriculum; and to generate aspirations for future careers. Packed with practical examples and handouts.

Steve Silberman (2015) *Neurotribes: The Legacy of Autism and How to Think Smarter about People Who Think Differently*

A social history of autism, addressing the origins of ableism in our culture, autism as a social justice issue and the potential for a more inclusive future.

Introduction to GLP

Gestalt Language Processing (GLP) is associated with autism and ADHD, but you can be a Gestalt Language Processor and not be autistic. Gestalt Language Processors acquire language by:

- Focusing on the intonational patterns of speech first.

- Processing the sound-stream as a 'whole', rather than segmented into words.

- Acquiring language in phrases and sentences, songs and scripts.

- Copying back the exact intonation pattern, volume, speed and even accent of a heard phrase.

- Associating these chunks of language with a particular situation, which encompasses the sensory experience or emotional nuance.

- The chunks of language are the soundtrack to an experience.

- Using these chunks of language later when there is an association with the original situation in which they heard the language chunk.

- Processing a whole experience: the sounds, sights, movements and feelings, and reproducing this 'whole' later.

The 'chunks' of language that we may hear a child produce are also known as delayed echolalia. Contrary to previous clinical assumptions, echolalia is NOT meaningless. It is rich in meaning for the child. The connection may not immediately be obvious to an unfamiliar listener, but attuned communication partners can 'do the detective work' to identify the likely intended meaning for an individual child (Prizant 1983).[1] It is vital for the child's communication development that these language wholes, also known as language 'gestalts' are recognised as meaningful communication.

Many GLPs are minimally speaking or have very unclear speech. There will be other signs that they are gestalt processors, such as:

- Reproducing a whole experience: acting it out or expecting it to be the same each time.

- Watching, rewinding and rewatching clips on tv or YouTube.

- If the child is vocalising, they may be reproducing the intonation patterns of speech they have heard.

- The child may have a love of music and song, and respond more to this than spoken language.

Gestalt Language Processors, when supported with the right strategies, progress predictably through the following stages of language acquisition (Blanc 2012[2]; Blanc et al 2023[3]):

The Stages of Natural Language Acquisition

		Examples
Stage 1	Language gestalts (wholes, scripts, songs, language soundtracks from experiences)	Zoom zoom zoom, we're going to the moon! It's a dinosaur!
Stage 2	Mitigations: a) Shortening long gestalts b) Dividing them into chunks c) Recombining different chunks	We're going to the moon! We're going We're going to the shops It's an octopus!
Stage 3	Isolated single words Word + word combinations of referential single words	dinosaur; rocket dinosaur . . . big; rocket . . . up
Stage 4	Original phrases and beginning sentences	We got dinosaur Put rocket up there
Stage 5	Original sentences with more complex grammar	I can get the dinosaurs I don't want to put my shoes on
Stage 6	Original sentences culminating in a complete grammar system	Who could have taken the dinosaurs? I've been looking for my shoes

Gestalt Language Processors require adults to model language in phrases (rather than single words) at the early stages of language acquisition. They are drawn to the musicality of language and are more likely to pick up a language gestalt if it is presented in a way they find interesting and enticing. This may be through song, or through phrases with rich musical intonation, a dramatic tone, an interesting rhythm or a fun voice.

If we only model single words, a Gestalt Language Processor is likely to get 'stuck' in their language development. They typically do not progress to combining their single words into two-word phrases. Their natural progression is to break a gestalt down into a shorter chunk, and then into the component words. If their 'gestalt' is a single word, this cannot be broken down, and so they cannot naturally progress in their language development. They just end up with a lot of single words.

By contrast when adults model whole phrases first, e.g. 'let's build a tower', 'we can throw the ball', the child acquires useful gestalts which can then start to be broken down into shorter chunks and then combined with new words or chunks, e.g. 'let's . . . throw the ball', 'we can . . . kick it'. This process of shortening of gestalts and 'mix-and-matching' then allows the child to isolate single words. This marks stage 3, where we see both single words and word + word combinations such as 'brick . . . tower' and 'brick . . . on'. Phrases and sentences with self-generated grammar will follow.

With the right language modelling, which is informed by knowledge of Gestalt Language Processing, children are likely to continue to acquire full advanced grammatical language with a wide vocabulary. If GLPs receive language intervention which has been designed for an Analytic Language Processor (the route whereby single words are acquired first), this is likely to be detrimental to their language development. They will not be able to naturally move through the stages described earlier.

With the Natural Language Acquisition framework (Blanc 2012, Blanc et al 2023), regular language samples are taken in order to track a child's progression. This ensures that appropriate language supports are used for the child's stage of language acquisition. This analysis needs to be carried out by a communication partner (usually a Speech and Language Therapist) who is familiar with the child's language.

The child needs to develop trust in the communication partner, in order to experiment with new language and move through the stages of language acquisition. In fact trust and connection are foundational for this approach. We don't prompt language or train compliance. We notice what the child loves to do, what kind of experiences and language they are drawn to, and we provide lots of opportunities to explore this. From this they show us their genuine communication intent, and they communicate naturally and spontaneously.

Notes

1 Prizant, B. (1983) 'Language acquisition and communicative behavior in autism: Toward an understanding of the "whole" of it' *Journal of Speech and Hearing Disorders* 48(3), 296–307.
2 Blanc, M. (2012) *Natural Language Acquisition on the Autism Spectrum: The Journey from Echolalia to Self-Generated Language* Madison, WI: Communication Development Center, Inc.
3 Blanc, M., Blackwell, A. & Elias, P. (2023) 'Using the natural language acquisition protocol to support Gestalt language development' *Perspectives of the ASHA Special Interest Groups*.

Stage 1 GLP language tracker

What the child said (if it was a long script, see if you can pick out a word or a section)	What might it mean? Where did you first hear it? Could it be from a video or song? Does it sound like it carries a strong emotion?

What the child said (if it was a long script, see if you can pick out a word or a section)	What might it mean? Where did you first hear it? Could it be from a video or song? Does it sound like it carries a strong emotion?

Language sample template

#	Speaker	Utterance	Context/Notes	Stage

#	Speaker	Utterance	Context/Notes	Stage

#	Speaker	Utterance	Context/Notes	Stage

#	Speaker	Utterance	Context/Notes	Stage

#	Speaker	Utterance	Context/Notes	Stage

#	Speaker	Utterance	Context/Notes	Stage

Total number of utterances	50	Percentages:
Stage 0		
Stage 1		
Stage 2		
Stage 3		
Stage 4		

Multi-modal (AAC) language sample template

Abbreviations for modality: sp (speech/mouth-words), cb (communication book/board), iPad (high-tech AAC) (or add your own, and specify the resources that the child used)

Add any other useful info about joint-referencing, proximity, showing, reaching, pointing, etc, under 'context/notes'.

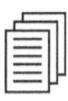

#	Speaker	Utterance	Context/Notes	Modality	Stage

#	Speaker	Utterance	Context/Notes	Modality	Stage

#	Speaker	Utterance	Context/Notes	Modality	Stage

#	Speaker	Utterance	Context/Notes	Modality	Stage

#	Speaker	Utterance	Context/Notes	Modality	Stage

#	Speaker	Utterance	Context/Notes	Modality	Stage

Total number of utterances	50	Percentages:	
Stage 0			
Stage 1			
Stage 2			
Stage 3			
Stage 4			

Stage 1 GLP: Examples of useful phrases

There is no set list: these are just to give you ideas

Sharing ideas	Look at that! Let's do it again! We need more Put it on Take it off
Shared joy	I love it! We did it! It's my favourite We're having fun That was the best
Describing objects, people or activities	It's dirty That was loud! Too hot! We're all wet!
Protesting	No way I'm not sure Don't do that Stop it
Transitioning	Let's go! Got to get ready In the car On the bus
Sensory regulation	Need to move Have to jump Find fidget toys
Self-advocacy	I can do it myself Give me space Need some quiet

Also consider songs that might accompany daily activities, e.g. getting dressed, brushing teeth, feeling hungry, having to wait, feeling worried and so on. The YouTube channels *Playtime with Tor*, *Cocomelon* and *Super Simple Songs* might provide inspiration!

Lines from favourite tv shows, movies or stories are also potentially helpful. Experiment with what appeals to your child.

Also consider using rich intonation, a musical tone, the pitch-range used by your child and fun voices.

Stage 1 GLP: Communication intentions inventory

Use this sheet to track a child's stage 1 gestalts by communication functions.

We're aiming for 2–3 phrases for each communication function.

This ensures that they have a good breadth of language for later stages.

Sharing ideas	
Shared joy	
Describing objects, people or activities	
Protesting	
Transitioning	
Sensory regulation	
Self-advocacy	
Others:	

Developmental sentence types

Adapted from Laura Lee (1966)

Nouns	Designators	Descriptive items	Verbs	Vocabulary items
ball, car, Mommy, kitty, hot dog, etc; **balls**, cars, men; me, something, nobody; book? car? truck?	here, there, this, that, it those, these this? that? here? there?	big, pretty, broken, one, two, more, on, off, up, none; my, his; red? big?	go! stop! wait! come! eat, sleep, walk, fell; eating, sleeping, ate, went; eat? sleep? can't, won't, won't?	here, there, this, that, it those, these this? that? here? there?
a ball, ball truck; more balls, Daddy ball; other truck; big car, dirty truck, baby bear; the cars car truck, Mommy Daddy; now car; doggie bone; car garage; Mommy window; this one, my truck, her cookie; not car, not truck, not this; another truck? which one? and this, and car	here car, that truck, it truck; there trucks; that again; there now; that one, here something; not this, not there, that truck? this car? who this? what that? and this, and here, and there	car broken, truck dirty, light off, tv on, car there, truck here; cars here, lights on; that pretty, it big, something here, another one; car broken? it gone? where car? what here? who there?	hit ball; sit chair; fall down; baby sleep, that go, it fall; saw car; eat cookies, sees cars; eat now, fall too; see it, find one; not fall, can't go; see it? go home? where go? what find? what take? who go? and sleeping; wanna go; gonna go	for Daddy, in car; on chairs, in cars; too big, all gone, up now, here again, right here, over there; to you, in it; not big, not here; in here? all gone? and big, but dirty, and here

Nouns	Designators	Descriptive items	Verbs	Vocabulary items
my big car; the car in front; all of them; some other cars; now the car; the car the truck; the car the garage; all of mine; not that one; the other car? which other one? How many cookies? and the car, car and truck	here another car; there another car; this a red car; it my truck; here some cars; here car now, there car now, there Mommy Daddy, that somebody car, here his car, that not car, that a car? who that boy? what that one? here and truck	the car broken, the tv on, car in garage; Spot a good dog; all cars broken; light off now; truck too dirty; it off now; this not broken; it off now? where that one? who in car? what colour car? car and truck here?	eat the cookie; put the table; take off hat, turn on light; the car go, a boy eat; goes in barn; see car now, got in too; want it now; not fall down; see that one? eat more cookies? where put car? what take out? what find here? what doing to car? and find car; wanna see it, gonna go home; gotta find it	dog, cow, pig, 1234; in the car, for the boy; on the chairs, in car too, back over there, on my head; not in it; in here too? in the car? and for me

Developmental sentence analysis

Reprinted from Laura Lee (1974)

Score	Indefinite pronouns or noun modifiers	Personal pronouns	Main verbs	Secondary verbs
1	it, this, that	1st & 2nd person: I, me, my, mine, you, your(s)	**A.** Uninflected verb: I *see* you. **B:** Copula, is or 's: It's red. **C:** is + verb + ing: He *is coming.*	
2		3rd person: he, him, his, she, her, hers	**A.** -s and –ed: *plays, played* **B:** Irregular past: *are, saw* **C:** Copula: *am, are, was, were* **D:** Auxiliary: *am, are, was, were*	Five early developing infinitives: I *wanna see.* (want *to see*) I'm *gonna see.* (going *to see*) I *gotta see.* (got *to see*) *Lemme* [to] see. (let me *[to] see*) *Let's* [to] play. (let [us *to*] *play*)
3	**A.** no, some, more, all, lot(s), one(s), two (etc.), other(s), another. **B.** something, somebody, someone	**A.** Plurals: we, us, our(s), they, them, their **B.** these, those		Non-complementing infinitives: I stopped *to play.* I'm afraid *to look.* It's hard *to do* that.
4	nothing, nobody, none, no one		**A.** can, will, may + verb: *may go* **B.** Obligatory do + verb: *don't go* **C.** Emphatic do + verb: I *do see*	Participle, present or past: I see a boy *running.* I found the toy *broken.*

Score	Indefinite pronouns or noun modifiers	Personal pronouns	Main verbs	Secondary verbs
5		Reflexives: myself, yourself, himself, herself, itself, themselves		**A.** Early infinitival complements with differing subjects in kernels: I want you *to come*, Let him *[to] see*. **B.** Later infinitival complements: I had *to go*, I told him *to go*, I tried *to go*, He ought *to go*. **C.** Obligatory deletions: Make it *[to] go*. **D.** Infinitive with wh-word: I know what *to get*, I know how *to do* it.
6		**A.** Wh- pronouns: who, which, whose, whom, what, that, how many, how much **B.** Wh- word + infinitives: I know *what to do*, I know *who(m) to take*.	**A.** could, would, should, might + verb: *might come, could be* **B.** Obligatory does, did + verb **C.** Emphatic does, did + verb	
7	**A.** any, anything, anybody, anyone **B.** every, everything, everybody, everyone **C.** both, few, many, each, several, most, least, much, next, first, last, second (etc.)	(his) own, one, oneself, whichever, whoever, whatever: Take *whatever* you like.	**A.** Passive with *get*, any tense Passive with *be*, any tense **B.** must, shall + verb: *must come* **C.** have + verb + en: *I've eaten.* **D.** have got: *I've got* it.	Passive infinitival complement: With *get*; I have *to get dressed*. I don't want to *get hurt.* With *be*: I want *to be pulled*, It's going to *be locked.*
8			**A.** have/had been + verb + ing **B.** modal + have + verb + en: *may have eaten* **C.** modal + be + verb + ing: *could be playing* **D.** Other auxiliary combinations: *should have been sleeping.*	Gerund: *Swinging* is fun. I like *fishing.*

Score	Negatives	Conjunctions	Interrogative reversals	Wh- questions
1	it, this, that + copula or auxiliary is, 's, + not: This *is not* a dog., That *is not* mine. It's *not* moving.		Reversal of copula: *Isn't it* red? *Were they* there?	
2				**A.** who, what, what + noun: *Who* am I? *What* is he eating? *What book* are you reading? **B.** where, how many, how much, what . . . do, what . . . for: *Where did* to go? *How much* do you want? *What* is he doing? *What* is a hammer *for?*
3		and		
4	can't, don't		Reversal of auxiliary be: *Is he* coming? *Isn't he* coming? *Was he* going?	
5	isn't, won't	**A.** but **B.** so, and so, so that **C.** or, if		When, how, how + adjective: *When* shall I come? *How* do you do it? *How big* is it?
6		because	**A.** Obligatory do, does, did: *Do they* run? *Does it* bite? *Didn't it* hurt? **B.** Reversal of modal: *Can you* play? *Won't it* hurt? *Shall I* sit down? **C.** Tag question: It's fun, *isn't it?* It isn't fun, *is it?*	

Score	Negatives	Conjunctions	Interrogative reversals	Wh- questions
7	All other negatives: **A.** Uncontracted negatives: I can *not go.* He has *not gone.* **B.** Pronoun-auxiliary or pronoun-copula contraction: I'm *not* coming. He's *not* here. **C.** Auxiliary-negative or copula-negative contraction: He *wasn't* going, He *hasn't* been seen, It *couldn't* be mine, They *aren't* big.			Why, what if, how come, how about + gerund: *Why* are you crying? *What if* I won't do it? *How come* he is crying? *How about* coming with me?
8		**A.** where, when, how, while, whether (or not), til, until, unless, since, before, after, for, as, as + adjective + as, as if, like, that, than: I know *where* you are, Don't come *til* I call. **B.** Obligatory deletions: I run faster *than* you [run], I'm *as big as* a man [is big], It looks *like* a dog [looks]. **C.** Elliptical deletions (score o): That's *why* [I took it], I know *how* [I can do it]. **D.** Wh- words + infinitive: I know *how* to do it. I know *where* to go.	**A.** Reversal of auxiliary have: *Has he* seen you? **B.** Reversal with two or three auxiliaries: *Has he* been eating? *Couldn't he have* waited? *Could he have been* crying? *Wouldn't he have been* going?	Whose, which, which + noun: *Whose* car is that? *Which book* do you want?

DSS Level 1 grammar constructions

Listen out for these in your child's natural language. Consider consciously using them, but only when they feel useful and natural.

Indefinite pronouns: We need **it**! **This** is fun **That** one's the best	**Personal pronouns:** **I** know Give those to **me** It's for **you** That's **mine!** This one's **yours** Here's **my** shoes There's **your** car!
Main verbs: I **see** you! (uninflected) It**'s** red; that **is** mine (copula) He **is** coming (is + verb-ing)	**Negatives:** It's **not** broken
Interrogative reversals: **Am I**? **Were they** there? (reversal of copula) Gym	

DSS Level 2 grammar constructions

Listen out for these in your child's natural language. Consider consciously using them, but only when they feel useful and natural.

Personal pronouns:	Main verbs:
She is drawing It's **her** book **He** hurt **his** foot that's **hers**	The girl **plays** (-s verb ending) The boy **looked** (-ed verb ending) The dog **saw** the cat; she **ate** it (irregular past) I **am** big! You**'re** here! She **was** fast; you **were** not (copula) I **am jumping**; You **are climbing** I **was singing**; you **were dancing** (auxiliary 'to be' + verb-ing)
Secondary verbs:	**Wh- questions:**
Five early developing infinitives: I **wanna** see I'm **gonna** get it I've **got to** go **Let me** see **Let's** play this	**What** is that? **What**'s he doing? **Who** is it? **What** are they doing? **Where** are they? **How many**? **How much**? **What**'s it for?

© 2025, *Gestalt Language Processing*, Alison Battye, Routledge

DSS Level 3 grammar constructions

Listen out for these in your child's natural language. Consider consciously using them, but only when they feel useful and natural.

Noun modifiers:	Plural personal pronouns:
No books	**We** got one!
Some toys	It's for **us**
More pieces	It's **our** game
All the animals	This one is **ours**
Lots of pieces	**They** came
The **other** one	I saw **them**
Another train	It's **their** car
Something's wrong	**These** are broken
Somebody's here	**Those** are mine
Someone's crying	
Secondary verbs:	**Conjunctions:**
I stopped **to read**	We got bananas **and** apples
I'm afraid **to climb**	They're running **and** jumping
(non-complementing infinitives (with another verb)	

DSS Level 4 grammar constructions

Listen out for these in your child's natural language. Consider consciously using them, but only when they feel useful and natural.

Noun modifiers:	Main verbs:
Nobody saw There's **nothing** in there There's **none** left! **No one** can touch it	We **can** build another one That one **will** fit It **may** go here I **do** have it!
Secondary verbs:	**Negatives:**
I see a girl **running** I found the toy **broken** (past or present participle)	I **can't** reach We **don't** have any more
Interrogative reversals:	
Is he coming? **Isn't she** coming? **Was he** going? (reversal of auxiliary 'to be')	

DSS Level 5 grammar constructions

Listen out for these in your child's natural language. Consider consciously using them, but only when they feel useful and natural.

Personal pronouns:	**Secondary verbs:**
I can do it **myself** Don't hurt **yourself** (Also **himself, herself, itself, themselves**)	I want **you to come** Let **them (to) come** Make **it (to) go** (early infinitive complements with different subjects) I **had to go** We **tried to tidy** up (later infinitive complements)
Negatives:	**Conjunctions:**
It **isn't** here It **won't** fit	I want this piece **but** it won't fit She's hungry **so** she needs lots We could choose red **or** blue spots We can go **if** there's time
Wh- questions:	
When will it be ready? **How** big is it?	

DSS Level 6 grammar constructions

Listen out for these in your child's natural language. Consider consciously using them, but only when they feel useful and natural.

Personal pronouns: **Who**'s that? **Which** one fits? **Whose** is this? **How many** do we need? **How much** should we get? I know **what** to do I know **who** to take (wh- words with infinitives)	**Secondary verbs:** We **could** go today I **should** tidy up They **might** come She **does** need the car I **did** go there! (obligatory 'do') I **do** love this! (emphatic 'do')
Conjunctions: We need to wear our coat **because** it's cold today	**Interrogative reversals:** **Do they** fit there? (obligatory 'do') **Can you** play piano? **Won't it** hurt? (reversal of modal) This is fun, **isn't it**? (tag questions)

DSS Level 7 grammar constructions

Listen out for these in your child's natural language. Consider consciously using them, but only when they feel useful and natural.

Modifiers: **Any, anything, anybody** **Every, everything, everybody** **Both, few, many** **First, next, last**	**Main verbs:** The ball **was thrown** The book **was written** (passive tense) They **must** come! We **shall** go. I**'ve eaten** (have + verb-en) We**'ve got** it (have got)
Secondary verbs: I don't want **to get** hurt They want **to be** picked (passive infinitival complement)	**Negatives:** They **aren't** that big He **wasn't** going to come (plus all other negatives)
Wh- questions: **Why** do we have to shower? **How come** there's no milk? **What if** we don't go to the party?	

DSS Level 8 grammar constructions

Listen out for these in your child's natural language. Consider consciously using them, but only when they feel useful and natural.

Main verbs:	Conjunctions:
She **has been** running They **may have** eaten I **could be playing** right now We **should have been** sleeping	(in subordinate clauses) How will I know **where** you'll be? Can you get bread **when** you're out? How will I know **who** she is? I don't know **whether** to do it or not We need to keep kneading **until** it feels stretchy. I can't let you go **unless** you tell me where you will be. We need to take the bus **before** we take the train. Brush your teeth **after** you've finished breakfast. It's not **as nice as** the red one. I'd like the chocolate **that** has nuts. I can jump higher **than** I can hop.
Secondary verbs: I am **waiting** Swinging is **fun** (gerund: verb used as a noun)	
Interrogative reversals: **Has he** seen you? **Have they** been eating? (reversal of auxiliary 'to have')	
Wh- questions: **Whose** car is that? **Which** book do you want?	

Sample GLP report

Name:

Dob:

Date of Report:

Background information

XXX is an autistic girl who attends XXX Primary School in reception class. XXX experiences differences with sensory regulation and language development. XXX is an affectionate, playful, focused and sensitive little girl. She loves being outdoors, playing with blocks and making intricate and carefully thought-out structures, making playscripts with monster toys, and painting, drawing and colouring. XXX shows an interest in letters and numbers, for example counting along with an adult and examining the dots on dice, joining in with phonics songs and actions in class, and playing with magnetic letters and stamps.

Sensory regulation

XXX experiences sensory regulation differences. We know that autistic people's sensory systems can be undersensitive or oversensitive, and that this varies from day to day.

XXX does not like light touch, and startles to this. In contrast, she finds firm touch and deep pressure to the joints calming, and this may help regulate XXX before she has to take part in a more challenging activity, e.g. walking down a busy corridor to get to lunch.

XXX will often clamber over objects and bump into people: this is a sign of her proprioceptive challenges and is not deliberate. XXX benefits from being barefoot where possible as this allows her to receive more sensory feedback about where her body is in space. Walking and climbing over obstacles is also very helpful.

XXX loves being outdoors and when given a choice, will play outdoors. Being outdoors is very regulating, as there is room to move around freely, getting vestibular and proprioceptive feedback from uneven walking surfaces, and being able to reach, climb and balance.

XXX requires regular movement breaks outdoors in her educational setting, in order to maintain her sensory regulation for learning and interacting.

XXX requires a sensory diet designed by an Occupational Therapist trained in sensory integration and carried out by a trained TA with sensory integration knowledge. This will enable XXX to be regulated to allow her to access the curriculum and interact with her peers and teaching staff.

Attention and listening

XXX makes good use of her peripheral vision and is able to attend to what's happening across the whole room. She often display 'covert attention', attending when she does not look like she is.[1] She is very adept at 'reading the room'. She is extremely sensitive to emotional resonances and dissonance. She tends to mirror an adult's dysregulation, and so it is important that adults are aware of what they are bringing to the situation.

XXX gets pleasure from close looking and from touching items to her face. This supports her sensory regulation and ability to attend.

XXX needs supporting adults to understand that her attention and listening looks different from neurotypical patterns of attention and listening. She needs to be able to move around when listening. She needs furniture that allows her to rock and wobble, e.g. a 'Zuma' chair.

XXX needs to be able to choose where to sit in order to access learning. For example, when the other children are sitting together on the carpet for literacy time, XXX needs to be able to choose whether to join them, or sit elsewhere in the room.

Cognitive processing style

XXX presents as a 'Gestalt Cognitive Processor'. This cognitive processing style is associated with autism. 'Gestalt' means 'whole'. Gestalt processors tend to think in whole experiences, gathering all the many details that contribute to a whole experience, including the sensory experiences and the emotional associations. Gestalt processors will tend to expect an experience to contain all the same elements as it previously did. They will often incorporate optional portions of an event into their 'plan' of what happens in a particular situation. For example, if they go to the doctors' and have their chest examined, a gestalt processor will expect this to happen every time and will likely lift up their shirt in anticipation.

Gestalt cognitive processors are excellent at recognising patterns and sequences, because they can process a lot of information all at once. They may be able to visually memorise a complex array of objects, pictures, letters or numbers.

This can manifest in distress if a pattern that they have created is disrupted, for example if they have laid out toy cars and someone moves one. This is analogous to us removing part of a favourite toy, like ripping off a teddy's ear. XXX enjoys constructing towers with bricks, dice and puzzle pieces. She analyses each piece, taking into consideration its size and shape. She does not accept suggestions because she has a clear plan of what she is trying to achieve.

XXX is likely to have enthusiasms which allow her to build detailed knowledge in particular areas (this is called 'monotropism' and is recognised as an autistic strength). **Adults should support XXX's learning by making use of these enthusiasms. She will be motivated to learn concepts in literacy, numeracy and across the curriculum if they are mapped onto her current interests.**

As a gestalt processor, XXX may struggle to acquire literacy with a synthetic phonics approach. She is likely to need a 'whole word' reading approach. Making use of whole texts and whole sentences related to special interests and enthusiasms is a good entry point into literacy. Learning spelling patterns through 'rime-and-onset' (word families) is likely to be more accessible than synthetic phonics. **Literacy instruction will need to take into consideration XXX's literacy learning style, be it via whole word learning or phonics. XXX may need help with reading for comprehension.**

Language learning style

XXX presents as a 'Gestalt Language Processor'. Gestalt Language Processing is associated with autism, but is not exclusive to autism. Gestalt Language Processors acquire language by:

- Focusing on the intonational patterns of speech first.

- Processing the sound-stream as an unanalysed 'whole', rather than segmented into words.

- Acquiring language in phrases and sentences, songs and scripts (rather than single words first).

- Copying back the exact intonation pattern, volume, speed and even accent of a heard phrase.

- Associating these chunks of language with a particular situation, which encompasses the sensory experience or emotional nuance.

- Using these chunks of language later when there is an association with the original situation in which they heard the language chunk.

These 'chunks' of language are also known as delayed echolalia. Contrary to previous clinical assumptions, echolalia is NOT meaningless. It is rich in meaning for the child. The connection may not immediately be obvious to an unfamiliar listener, but attuned communication partners can 'do the detective work' to identify the likely intended meaning for an individual child (Prizant 1983, 48, 296–307).[2] It is vital for the child's communication development that these language wholes, also known as 'language gestalts' are recognised as meaningful communication.

Gestalt Language Processors, when supported with the right strategies, progress predictably through the following stages of language acquisition (Blanc 2012,[3] Blanc et al 2023[4])

The Stages of Natural Language Acquisition

		Examples
Stage 1	Language gestalts (wholes, scripts, songs and language of episodes	Zoom zoom zoom, we're going to the moon! It's a dinosaur!
Stage 2	Mitigations (mitigated gestalts and partial scripts) Mix-and-match combinations of partial scripts	We're going to the moon! We're going! We're going to the shops! It's an octopus!
Stage 3	Isolated single words Two-word combinations of referential single words	dinosaur; rocket dinosaur. . . big; rocket. . . up
Stage 4	Original phrases and beginning sentences	
Stage 5	Original sentences with more complex grammar	I can get the dinosaurs I don't want to put my shoes on
Stage 6	Original sentences using a complete grammar system	Who could have taken the dinosaurs? I've been looking for my shoes

Gestalt Language Processors require adults to model language in phrases (rather than single words) at the early stages of language acquisition. If we only model single words, a Gestalt Language Processor is likely to get 'stuck' at this single word stage. They typically do not progress to combining their single words into two-word phrases. By contrast when adults model whole phrases first, e.g. 'let's build a tower', 'we can throw the ball', the child can acquire useful gestalts which can then start to be broken down into stage 2 mitigations, e.g. 'let's get in the car', 'we can catch the ball'. Because of this 'mix-and-matching' of mitigated gestalts in stage 2, the child can then 'release' the single words. This marks stage 3, where we finally see both single words and two-word combinations such as 'brick tower' and 'brick on'. This is the start of self-generated language, and it naturally leads into stage 4, beginning sentences.

XXX has naturally acquired a lot of longer scripts from her favourite tv shows like 'Daniel Tiger' and 'Peppa Pig'. She quietly recites these as she is playing, and associations are made between what she is doing and what she has experienced in these shows. XXX's scripts are often very long (she has an excellent memory), but there might be a part where she gets louder and more emphatic: this is the part that she wants to communicate. We can sometimes pick put little bits of these scripts, like 'ok, George, open your eyes!' XXX's motor speech development is still immature, but so long as her natural speech is honoured and listened to, she will continue to get more accurate with her speech sounds, and we will more easily be able to identify her phrases. XXX's gestalts often involve physical movement in addition to the words. Whilst the intonation pattern is probably the aspect of the script that XXX is most proficient at reproducing (she is very musical), she is also able to use an increasing repertoire of consonants and vowels in her scripts. She also incorporates the vocal quality from the original sound source, speaking in the voice of the character.

XXX's scripts should be listened to, acknowledged and treated as meaningful. It can be hard to work out the connection as the meaning of the scripts are not literal. XXX's parents are crucial collaborators who help us to identify the source of new scripts.

Music is also a very strong modality for XXX, and she is acquiring a lot of favourite songs. Songs are very helpful for stage 2 mitigations as we can swop in other lines. For example, in 'Old Macdonald' we can change the animal, and in 'This is the way we wash our hands' we can swop in different actions.

The next step for XXX is to acquire shorter, more mitigable stage 1 gestalts. I have provided home and school with a GLP-friendly communication book. This is divided into communication intentions, with phrases for 'expressing ideas', 'shared joy', 'describing', 'transitions', 'regulation', 'self-advocacy' and 'my scripts'. Examples of these phrases are 'let's go', 'let's get another one', 'it's too noisy' and 'I need to move'.

With GLP intervention, XXX has acquired more useful, mitigable gestalts, such as 'come on', 'there you go', 'I don't want to', 'don't do that', 'go away' and 'what's next?' XXX is also acquiring some single words, such as 'carrot', 'potato', 'orange', 'purple' and 'storytime'. She will not naturally be able to build these into two-word phrases until she has more stage 1 and stage 2 language. She needs more phrases, rather than single words. Our work is to continue modelling useful stage 1 language. When XXX has around 50 useful mitigable gestalts, she is likely to naturally move into stage 2 and start 'mix-and-matching' her phrases to create new novel utterances.

With the right language modelling, which is informed by knowledge of Gestalt Language Processing, XXX is likely to continue to acquire self-generated language to cover a range of communication intentions. Just from stage 2 language, a child is able to use language more flexibly with a wider range of communication partners.

If XXX receives language intervention which has been designed for an Analytic Language Processor (the route whereby single words are acquired first), this is likely to be detrimental to her language development, and she will retreat into earlier stages of language acquisition.

It is very important that XXX is not exposed to prompted or prescribed language activities. This is counter-productive to the acquisition of self-generated language. Such techniques as sentence completion and cloze procedures do not lead to generalisation for Gestalt Language Processors. PECS is no longer considered an appropriate intervention for autistic children: its scope is far too limited, offering only phrases for requesting. There is more to language than requesting, and XXX is capable of expressing a wide range of communication intentions to meet her need for connection and to reflect her complex thought processes and profound understanding of emotions.

With the Natural Language Acquisition framework (Blanc 2012, Blanc et al 2023), regular language samples are taken in order to track a child's progression. This ensures that appropriate language modelling strategies are used for the child's stage of language acquisition. In order to accurately analyse language samples, the communication partner needs to be familiar with the child's language in order to recognise stage 1, 2, 3 or 4 language for this individual child. The child needs to develop trust in the communication partner, in order to experiment with new language and move through the stages of language acquisition.

XXX requires teaching staff to be trained in the basics of Gestalt Language Processing, so that they model language appropriate to his stage of language acquisition throughout the day and across the curriculum.

A Speech and Language Therapist who has received training in Gestalt Language Processing and Natural Language Acquisition should provide regular weekly therapy sessions which are child-led and play-based in order to model appropriate language and to track XXX's progression through the stages of GLP Natural Language Acquisition. The Speech and Language Therapist will need to advise on the content of XXX's GLP-friendly communication book.

XXX may in the future benefit from a communication app on an iPad which mirrors the content of her communication book. Autistic people report that when they are dysregulated it can be difficult for them to access their speech, and so having the opportunity to use alternative communication methods (a symbolised vocabulary package or text-to-speech) gives them another option. A Speech and Language Therapist will need to advise on this.

XXX needs the following from her school provision

- XXX needs supporting adults to understand that her attention and listening looks different from neurotypical patterns of attention and listening. She needs to be able to move around when listening. She needs furniture that allows her to rock and wobble, e.g. a 'Zuma' chair.

- XXX needs to be able to choose where to sit in order to access learning. For example, when the other children are sitting together on the carpet for literacy time, XXX needs to be able to choose whether to join them, or sit elsewhere in the room. A sensory diet designed by an Occupational Therapist and carried out by a trained TA with sensory integration knowledge will help to regulate her for learning and interacting.

- XXX needs regular movement breaks (at least twice a day, plus as needed if she is dysregulated) outdoors in her educational setting, in order to maintain her sensory regulation for learning and interacting.

- XXX needs a modified curriculum that incorporates her interests and enthusiasms. She will be motivated to learn concepts in literacy, numeracy and across the curriculum if they are mapped onto her interests.

- XXX needs literacy instruction which is matched to her literacy learning style, be it via whole word learning or analytic phonics.

- If XXX receives language intervention which has been designed for an Analytic Language Processor (the route whereby single words are acquired first), this is likely to be detrimental to her language development, and she will retreat to earlier stages of language acquisition.

- XXX requires teaching staff who are trained in the basics of Gestalt Language Processing, so that they model language appropriate to her stage of language acquisition throughout the day and across the curriculum.

- XXX needs Gestalt Language Modelling to be used in all activities, including all teaching activities. We use language to match what is happening, describing what we see, and what the child is doing and thinking.

- For Gestalt Language Processors, we avoid eliciting language. We don't probe, prompt or require a response. GLPs find questions very confusing until they are securely in stage 4 of Natural Language Acquisition. Until then, we teach by modelling language and behaviour, using invitational language like 'let's try squeezing it' or 'we can push this button'.

XXX needs the following Speech and Language Therapy provision

- A Speech and Language Therapist who has received training in Gestalt Language Processing and Natural Language Acquisition should provide regular weekly therapy sessions which are child-led and play-based in order to model appropriate language and to track XXX's progression through the stages of GLP Natural Language Acquisition (38 hours per academic year).

- The GLP-trained SLT needs regular time with teaching staff to update them about XXX's language acquisition. This should be incorporated into the weekly therapy sessions as described earlier. I recommend 45 minutes for the therapy session and 15 minutes for analysing the language sample and feeding back to staff each week.

- The GLP-trained SLT needs to provide an updated report for the annual review (1.5 hours once per year), and to attend termly meeting with the team around XXX (one hour six times per year).

- The total number of hours required is 45.5 hours per academic year.

- XXX may in the future benefit from a communication app on an iPad which mirrors the content of her communication book. Autistic people report that when they are dysregulated it can be difficult for them to access their speech, and so having the opportunity to use alternative communication methods (a symbolised vocabulary package or text-to-speech) gives them another option. A Speech and Language Therapist will need to advise on this.

Short-term goals (to end of year R)

1. XXX will continue to acquire new mitigable stage 1 language gestalts to cover a range of communication intentions, e.g. expressing ideas, expressing joy, describing, managing transitions, protesting, expressing sensory experiences, self-advocacy.

2. XXX will have access to a GLP friendly communication book, and adults will model a range of phrases from this, to match XXX's perceived communication desires. Adults should model phrases in all activities through the day, with at least 50 phrases being modelled in the school day.

The desired communication and interaction outcomes by the end of key-stage 1

- By the end of key-stage 1, XXX will be moving into stage 2 of Natural Language Acquisition and will be using mix-and-match phrases to communicate a range of communication intentions.

Notes

1 Gernsbacher, M. A., Stevenson, J. L., Khandakar, S. & Goldsmith, H. H. (2008, April) 'Why does joint attention look atypical in autism?' *Child Development Perspectives* 2(1), 38–45.
2 Prizant, B. (1983, September) 'Language acquisition and communicative behavior in autism: Toward an understanding of the "whole" of It' *Journal of Speech and Hearing Disorders*.
3 Blanc, M. (2012) 'Communication Development Center' *Natural Language Acquisition on the Autism Spectrum: The Journey from Echolalia to Self-Generated Language*.
4 Blanc, M., Blackwell, A. & Elias, P. (2023) 'Using the natural language acquisition protocol to support Gestalt language development' *Perspectives of the ASHA Special Interest Groups*.

Sample GLP AAC report

Name:

Dob:

Date of Report:

Background information

XXX has a diagnosis of autism and is currently minimally speaking. His parents contacted me about therapy to support his multi-modal communication.

XXX is an intentional communicator, who uses multi-modal (Total) communication, which includes vocalisations, gestures, body proximity, body movements, facial expressions and, more recently, a symbolised vocabulary package on an iPad. This is a form of Augmentative and Alternative Communication (AAC). XXX also uses YouTube video clips communicatively to share his thoughts and ideas, and to explore phrases that he finds interesting and appealing.

XXX shows signs of being a Gestalt Language Processor (GLP). He is attracted to whole phrases and the rich intonation of connected speech. He really enjoys funny voices and regional accents, and responds with smiles and laughter to familiar phrases that retain the voice quality of the original media source.

Like many minimally speaking autistic children, XXX has dyspraxia of speech. He struggles to initiate his voice, though he can access it when he is laughing, when he is engaged in high energy activities (dancing, bouncing, swinging, rolling) and when he is enjoying an activity.

XXX's Voco Chat package on his iPad allows him to access a range of communication intentions, including sharing ideas, expressing shared joy, describing, protesting, managing transitions, expressing sensory regulation needs and self-advocating. It is essential for his wellbeing and sense of community that XXX is able to share these communication intentions with others.

Current communication

Once he has established a trusting relationship with a familiar adult, XXX is keen to communicate using his multi-modal communication. He enjoys action songs, physical and sensory play (e.g. rocking or rolling or being squashed or wobbled on a peanut ball), sharing his favourite YouTube clips, and more recently, looking at a book together. He is especially engaged with a Lego Ideas book.

Adults are modelling phrases on his Voco Chat package to match his likely communication intention. For example, when he is laughing and vocalising during play on the peanut ball, we model 'I like it' and 'we're having fun!' When we play with a sensory toy and XXX wants to repeat this, we model 'let's do it again' and 'I need more'.

XXX has recently begun to press buttons on his Voco Chat package. He has recently said 'I'm so happy' and 'I love you', 'let's go' and 'I need to move'. He uses all of the 'my scripts' buttons which have been programmed with his favourite lines from YouTube clips. These express a range of communication intentions. For example, 'you can be my partner' to indicate he is enjoying being with someone; 'Mummy, Daddy, it's Christmas!' to indicate excitement about an upcoming event, 'don't make a mess, Daddy!' to indicate that something has gone wrong. He is also using his Voco Chat to request specific food items and activities. XXX is also enjoying looking at a book and having an adult model language around this book on his Voco Chat package.

XXX's vocalisations have increased since we started really listening out for them and repeating them back, and assuming that they were a word or phrase if they sound like a word or phrase. XXX has responded to this by vocalising more. His sound repertoire has expanded from just the /y/ sound to many more sounds. These are now said in tuneful syllables with varied consonants and vowels, e.g. [ayeyeyeye], [bibimamama]. XXX has also made attempts that sound very much like 'again' and 'I like it'.

XXX needs the following from his school provision

- **Adults need to model phrases on XXX's iPad as he accesses a full range of activities in school. They should use the 'My phrases' pages initially, using the different pages that have been set up around 'Sharing Ideas', 'shared joy', 'describing', 'protesting', 'transitions', 'regulation' and 'self-advocacy'. Adults need to model these phrases to match XXX's likely communication intention. For example, when he wants to do something again, we model 'Let's do it again' and 'I want to do it' and 'I need some more'. When he is upset, we model 'I don't like it', 'that's not right' or 'stop that'.**

- **Adults need to use the Voco Chat package during other activities like reading books, singing songs and watching videos. Adults should use the 'My phrases' pages and also the 'I want', 'play something' and 'do something'** pages. These pages are designed with phrases that naturally arise from activities like blowing bubbles, playing with a ball, with cars, building and so on. Adults should model phrases like 'it's my turn', 'pop it', 'blow a big bubble' and so on.

- XXX needs to be exposed to a wide range of language in a variety of situations. He will need to hear phrases many times in order to process them, and to learn the locations on his Voco Chat package. Initially we need to navigate to the right page and then model phrases. XXX should also be encouraged to just explore buttons by pressing them and hearing the message. This will help him learn what they mean.

- Teaching staff need to ensure that XXX can reach his iPad during class activities. The only exceptions are outdoor play or wet play.

- It is not enough to put an AAC system in front of a child and expect them to start using it. They are effectively learning a new language. Speaking children hear spoken language throughout the day every day. AAC-using children need to see and hear AAC language throughout the day every day.[1]

- Adults need to model 200 phrases per day, in order to model a range of language structures and communication intentions.[2] This is not as difficult as it sounds, as one interaction with a child can easily use ten modelled phrases. We are aiming for 'little and often' throughout the day.

- Adults need to be ready to respond to XXX's communication attempts on his AAC (and other modalities, e.g. speech). Every communication attempt should be treated as meaningful and important. Adults should use the current context to try to understand what XXX may be trying to convey, e.g. he is making an observation, he is wanting to share the moment, etc.

- XXX needs access to a range of play experiences, including large motor play, e.g. bouncing on a trampoline or peanut ball, running or jumping or dancing, playing with noise-makers, singing songs and looking at a favourite book. The adult should notice XXX's responses and model spoken language and language on his iPad to match his communication intentions, e.g. 'Look at this!', 'I love it!', 'what's next?' and 'need to move'.

- Adults should listen for all of XXX's attempts to vocalise and make words. If he says a word or a word-like utterance, adults should shape this into a word or phrase to match his intentions. For example, if he is dancing and laughing and vocalises something that sounds like 'yeah yeah yeah!' the adult should say 'yeah! I love this!'

XXX needs the following Speech and Language Therapy provision

- A Speech and Language Therapist who has received training in Gestalt Language Processing and Natural Language Acquisition to have oversight of his communication needs, including making edits to his AAC and liaising regularly with teaching staff.

- Regular weekly one-to-one therapy sessions with the GLP-trained SLT of 45 minutes' each plus 15 minutes liaison time with teaching staff and note-writing time (36 hours per year).

- Ten one-to-one therapy sessions with the GLP-trained SLT and parents during school holidays, to ensure that the AAC system meets XXX's social and educational needs across contexts (ten hours per year).

- The GLP-trained SLT needs to liaise with the school staff, to ensure a joined-up approach to communication and AAC (6 hours per year).

- The GLP-trained SLT will need to make regular edits to XXX's Voco Chat package to ensure that it allows his language to grow with his interests and preferences, and so that the language is structured appropriately for his GLP needs (ten hours per year).

- The GLP-trained SLT needs to provide an updated report for the annual review (three hours once per year), and to attend the annual review meeting (two hours per year).

- The total number of hours required is 67 hours per year.

Communication goals to the next annual review (April 2024)

1. XXX will have a repertoire of at least 20 different phrases on his Voco Chat package on the iPad, which he uses regularly to express at least three different communication intentions (e.g. expressing joy, protesting, self-advocacy).

2. XXX will explore his Voco Chat package with an adult in a range of different activities at school, e.g. looking at a book, playing with sensory toys, when engaged in movement activities. He will show engagement by looking, listening or pressing buttons on Voco Chat in a communicative context.

3. XXX will expand his vocalisations, so that he produces a variety of different consonants and vowels in syllable strings. XXX will use consonants including approximants /y w l/, nasals /m n; and fricatives /f s sh/.

Notes

1 Battye, A. (2018) *Who's Afraid of AAC? The UK Guide to Augmentative and Alternative Communication* Routledge Speechmark, pp. 126–133.
2 Caufield, F. & Carrillo, D. (2011, December 1) '200 a day the easy way: Putting it in practice' *Perspectives on Augmentative and Alternative Communication* 20(4), 125–133.

Index

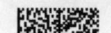